ER DOC

Defining Moments
of a Career in
Emergency Medicine

Reggie Duling, M.D.

Some names and identifying details have been changed to protect the privacy of individuals.

ISBN: 9798694076494

To Janina, for your love and support, for making me a better person, for the joy and laughter, and for giving me everything that matters in this life. I love you forever.

To Logan, Carson and Jessica, for being my inspiration, for the love, giggles and hugs, and for the joy of watching you become the amazing people you are. I love you with all my heart.

To my mom and dad, Diane and Bill, for your unconditional love, and for teaching me many of life's most important lessons. I love you so much and will always appreciate everything you have done for me.

To Ruth and Randy, for giving me a family I cherish every day, for your love and support, and for creating the most incredible woman I have ever known. I love you dearly.

To my family in WA, OH, MI and TN, for your love, encouragement, and open arms. I love you.

To all my friends, for your love and friendship, your generosity of spirit, and for the countless warm memories. I love you all.

TABLE OF CONTENTS

Introduction

The ER is an amazing place, where within a few short hours one can witness all that defines human existence: the unfortunate and unseemly consequences of the self-destructive nature of human beings, the coexistence of an indefatigable will to live, laughter that comes from the most unexpected sources and fills your soul, and horrific and unspeakable suffering and tragedy.

Working as an ER doctor can be hilarious, ironic, devastating, emotionally draining, and more monotonous than most people would think, but it's rarely boring.

If you remember the TV show "ER" and always wondered how realistic it was, I would put it like this: it was almost always true to life, but the producers packed about a month's worth of the most interesting cases into one hour.

I hope this book gives you a feel for some of what goes on in emergency departments across the country, 24 hours a day. These are the stories that have affected me most during my more than two decades on the front lines of the American health care system.

I thought about including chapters whining about our difficult work environment in the ER, but honestly, who would want to read it? You are probably reading a book to escape from your own problems and find some inner peace. Why read about someone else who thinks he has it bad? Is there such a thing as a stress-free job, especially one which deals with the public?

Sure, I could tell you how the electronic medical record drives us all insane. Studies have shown that an ER doc makes over 4,000 mouse clicks during a typical shift, and that we spend over half our time on the computer.

I could list some of my pet peeves, like when I ask a patient who is covered with a blanket to point to where their stomach hurts only to have them move their hand around *under* the blanket and say, "Right here." If my x-ray vision worked through blankets, it would probably see through skin, and I wouldn't have to ask where it hurt.

Or how laying in a bed paralyzes some people. I'm not talking about being unable to make a decision, aka paralysis of analysis, or merely being overwhelmed. I'm talking about being physically paralyzed, as in I ask the patient to wiggle their toes or lift their leg off the bed, and the patient says they can't do it. I saw you walk into the ER. You walked back to the room. You climbed into the bed. Now I ask you to lift your leg and you are apparently so weak you can't even get your foot off the bed? Doctors are smart enough to know that those findings are inconsistent. No one loses that much strength by becoming supine.

I might point out things that gross me out, like when a toddler throws his pacifier on the floor and his mom picks it up and puts it right back in his mouth. *Off the floor in an ER*? Ewwww! I'm a big fan of the 5-second rule, but it does *not* apply in the ER.

My wife could tell you about how being an ER doctor ruins watching any TV show with a medical storyline. OK, maybe not *every* ER doctor does this, but I do. I'm the reason we don't watch Grey's Anatomy anymore. Once, a contestant on The Bachelorette injured his *finger* and was transported by ambulance "lights and sirens" to the ER on a cardiac monitor! Come on, man. Lights and sirens? Really? Ever heard of a splint and having a friend drive you to the ER? If you think this is insensitive, you might want to skip the chapter titled "You're a Man, Right?"

For that matter, I'm probably not much better to watch sports with. I find it amusing what announcers think qualifies as a "tough-it-out" performance. First, let's not compare any of our most popular sports like football, basketball and baseball to actual tough-guy sports. Any man or woman who has stepped into the Octagon is, by default, tougher than anyone who has ever run onto a baseball diamond. To my point, want to know my professional, ER doctor opinion on the most overrated "tough guy performance" in sports history? Hands down it was Curt Schilling's "bloody sock" game. I'm not saying his surgery, rehab, recovery—whatever it took for him to return from injury—weren't difficult. But throwing a ball after losing maybe ten red blood cells? I've lost more blood shaving. Google Clint Malarchuk, the NHL player who took a skate to the neck and lacerated his carotid artery. He could have bled to death right on the ice. *That's* a sports injury an ER doctor sees and goes "Holy. Shit." Michael Jordan's flu game? Badass. Curt Schilling? The camera kept zooming in on his sock like it was the Shroud of Turin. Please.

And yes, I understand that in the last two paragraphs I threw shade at a potential future Hall of Fame pitcher while openly admitting that I watch The Bachelorette.

I'm an overweight, balding man in my 50's. I gave up any pretense of being studly years ago when I traded my Mustang in on a minivan. For any men who haven't yet experienced that rite of passage, prepare yourselves, because it's a tough day. The salesman stood by my side, watching my Mustang being driven into the dealership, shaking his head in empathy.

He quietly said, "I'm sorry for your loss. A lot of guys say they'd give their left nut to own a Mustang. Think of owning a minivan as the same thing, except you have to give them both up." He consoled me by throwing in what he called their "bereavement package" which included a cigar and two tickets to a Mariners game. He then offered this advice, "I say this as a friend. If you're smart, do NOT smoke the cigar in the minivan."

You know you've hit domesticated middle age clinging to vestiges of classic male behavior when you kindly ask your wife, "Hey, babe, can you bring me a beer? Dancing With The Stars is on." I still call 'em like I see 'em.

I'm also known for having a knack for saying the absolute wrong thing at the worst possible time. I once told a patient she was pregnant when she clearly wasn't expecting the news. Awkwardly trying to further the conversation after she didn't respond, I continued, "I bet you didn't see that coming." She replied, "Well, no, I'm blind." It's a gift. Just ask my wife.

I ask in advance for forgiveness if things I find funny don't really tickle your funny bone. I realized long ago that my sense of humor sometimes doesn't suit "normal" people whose behavior is more socially acceptable. I still chuckle when a heavily tattooed IV drug user screams as I inject an abscess that he "hates needles."

I still roll my eyes when I tell a patient I need to do a rectal exam, meaning stick my finger in their butt, and they ask in a way that does not seem rhetorical, "Isn't there another way to check that?" If there were, don't you think I would choose that option? I want to say, "Of course there is, but how else was I going to be able to put my finger in your ass? If I were doing this for medical reasons, I'd be wearing gloves!"

I also apologize for any defensiveness you might perceive. ER doctors definitely feel persecuted at times, as we catch grief from all sides. I know how hard it is to do this job, and I have incredible respect and admiration for those who do it.

I hope you will indulge some of our peccadillos and superstitions in the ER. I don't believe in all of them, but I do enjoy them. On a rational level, I don't really believe that a full moon causes weird things to happen, or cosmically forces strange people to come to the ER, but have I ever been at work and wondered aloud, "Is it a full moon tonight?" Yes, I have.

You will find no shortage of books with "true stories from the ER" or similarly themed titles on Amazon or in your local bookstore (which these days is also usually an Amazon store). Better writers, smarter doctors, and ER professionals around the country have put pen to paper, or fingers to keyboards, to document their stories for your consideration and entertainment. I am sure I am not alone in the feeling that I *needed* to write this book. You may have read other stories from the ER, but you haven't read these, because they are mine. I would like to share them, perhaps partly as a form of catharsis, as I've been carrying some of them around for over two decades.

More than anything, though, what I hope to convey in this book is the humanity inexorably linked to the practice of emergency medicine. We see some patients and families on their worst days. At times, the public sees us on ours. It is a privilege I do not take for granted to be able to share this thing we call life with each other on such a human level in the ER.

The experience of working in the ER is humbling. I can tell you that there are few experiences more exhilarating than knowing that you played a pivotal role in saving a life. I can also disclose that there are few responsibilities more solemn than being trusted with the life of another human being. When things don't go as planned, one can't help but ruminate over whether you missed something or failed to pick up on an important clue. Self-doubt is disruptive to one's psyche, confidence, self-esteem and sleep patterns.

In these pages I have tried to examine my journey and those whose lives are forever intertwined in it. This is an exploration of how a career choice made 25 years ago has affected my life so profoundly. I can only tell this story from my perspective. I know dozens of anecdotes you'd be fascinated to hear that aren't mine to tell. Get a group of ER docs together and you might hear many tales more compelling than those I describe herein.

These are my stories, random thoughts and philosophies, presented in no particular order. I hope you are as entertained, moved and inspired by them as I have been. While I wish to peel back the curtain a bit, I hope one message is clear: I love being an ER doc. This is an insight into the ER, a sometimes magical, sometimes medieval place where, when you boil it all down, only two things happen: life and death. I know something about both.

CHAPTER ONE

My First Night On Call

As my alarm clock began blasting the full-length rendition of Free Bird, I knew it was going to be a great day. You see, I'm a rock and roller. Sadly, my teenage years coincided with disco and early 80's trash, but thanks to FM 104.7, WIOT, the classic rock station in my hometown of Toledo, Ohio, I grew up on a steady diet of "getting the Led out," RUSH, AC/DC, Pink Floyd and Jimi Hendrix, among many others.

It took me nearly ten minutes to roll out of the rack, in part because it was 5 a.m., a ridiculously early time to wake up, and partly because I jammed along with Lynyrd Skynyrd, alternating between air guitar and air piano. During the pause for station identification, I realized that was the day I would start my third year of medical school.

The first two years of medical school had been the easiest of my adult life, which is still true to this day. After nearly four years of Active Duty in the Army followed by finishing college in three years while working part-time loading trucks at UPS from 11 p.m. to 3 a.m. five days a week while continuing to serve in the Army Reserve and National Guard, two years of reading books had seemed pretty chill in comparison.

That's not to say medical school is easy; it isn't. Neither is working 50 hours a week in a factory in a job you can't stand so that you can support your family. Nor is serving your country overseas to defend our American way of life. It all depends on your scale of difficulty. If you were smart enough to get into medical school, high school probably wasn't that challenging for you. If you next went to college and partied your ass off for four years, then yes, medical school was probably a rude awakening, but anyone who's worked for a living wouldn't bat an eye, at least initially.

My third year of medical school would begin with my first clinical rotation on the Cardiology IV service. There were five cardiology services, with Cardiology V reserved for heart transplant patients.

After spending the first two years of medical school reading about seemingly abstract diseases and treatments, it was a nice change of pace to be on the wards.

The cardiology service was where I would learn about congestive heart failure, acute myocardial infarction, cardiac transplantation, cardiac medications, and nearly everything else related to the heart.

Just before 6 a.m., I found the nursing station on the cardiology floor. I knew I was in the right place when I saw a few classmates milling around, all of us in our new, pressed, short white coats. Right at six, Jim showed up. Jim was an intern in the Department of Internal Medicine. He was smart as a whip, but more impressive was the way he seemed to know what was important and what wasn't. He was the classic "see the forest for the trees" guy. Internists memorize tons of facts, the kind most of us forget within a few years of medical school, but which internists seem to retain forever. There's a saying in medicine, "When you hear hoofbeats, think horses, not zebras." In other words, there are a lot more horses around than zebras. Common things happen commonly. A dry mouth is much more likely to indicate dehydration, perhaps as a sign of diabetes, than it is to indicate

Sjogren's syndrome. Diabetes is a horse; Sjogren's is a zebra. Internists are the ultimate zebra hunters. That's why internists are so important and valued. When you hear hoofbeats and there's not a horse in sight, you need someone who can spot a zebra. While he seemed to know a zebra when he saw one, Jim was focused on the horses. He also possessed a characteristic every bit as important as medical knowledge in surviving internship: efficiency.

My first day of cardiology also introduced me to Dr. Don Charlton, the attending cardiologist on Cardiology IV. Dr. Charlton had one distinguishing feature that you couldn't help but notice: when he spoke, it sounded like he had a severe case of laryngitis. He strained to speak loudly enough so that others could hear him. When I first introduced myself to Dr. Charlton, I was surprised to hear his raspy voice, but was smart enough to just shut up and listen, unlike one of my classmates who couldn't help but note, "Sounds like you have a bad cold there." If I had anything going for me, it was the little voice in my head that told me Dr. Charlton didn't have a cold. Call it instinct or gut feeling, but over the years I have learned to trust that little voice.

At 5 a.m. the next morning I began the second day of the rotation, which would be my first night taking call. Being on call meant you didn't get to leave; you stayed in the hospital overnight to handle any problems that might arise and admit any new patients to the service. As luck would have it, I would spend my first night on call with Jim. We spent much of it outside the room of Mr. Robert Zimmerman.

Mr. Zimmerman had a habit of going into v-tach, or ventricular tachycardia. V-tach is divided into two clinical entities: v-tach with a pulse, and v-tach without a pulse. If you had a pulse but were having chest pain, shortness of breath, or were unable to sustain adequate blood pressure, you were considered unstable. Pulseless v-tach and unstable v-tach were treated with electricity; what was affectionately referred to as "Edison medicine."

Mr. Zimmerman maintained a pulse during his episodes of v-tach, but his blood pressure dropped and he developed chest pain, making him unstable. He was being treated with a new drug, amiodarone, which the cardiologist hoped would stabilize his heart rhythm. He was also scheduled to have an implantable defibrillator placed in his chest, a device that would shock his heart back into a normal rhythm and prevent him from dropping dead once he left the hospital.

In the meantime, Jim and I diligently listened for an alarm from the patient's monitor as we finished up the H&P's (histories and physicals) on the patients admitted to the service that day. Mr. Zimmerman's monitor would alarm as he experienced another episode of v-tach. Jim would run in the room, give him 50 milligrams of methohexital to ensure that Mr. Zimmerman wouldn't feel anything, then he'd grab the paddles of the defibrillator, put them on Mr. Zimmerman's chest, and "KER-CHUNK!", his chest would heave as the electrical shock cardioverted him back into a normal rhythm. Jim made it look easy. After seeing this ritual performed a couple of times, I was watching intently when Jim asked me, "How much Brevital do you want to give him?"

"50 milligrams," I responded, having heard him give the order twice already.

"Good." Jim seemed pleased. It wasn't brain surgery, and Jim probably wasn't happy that I knew the dose so much as it showed that at least I paid attention. Paying attention is crucial in medicine.

Jim handed me the paddles and said, "Go for it."

Hesitant at first, I was suddenly excited. I had been on the wards for two days and I was already shocking someone! This was one of the reasons I had gone to medical school. As a kid I loved watching "Emergency!"

No matter what happened to someone on that show, it seemed they were always defibrillated. You could have an ingrown toenail and the next thing you knew someone was yelling, "Clear!"

We were trained to use the defibrillator as part of Advanced Cardiac Life Support, or ACLS, before beginning our third year, but it was much more exhilarating doing it on a live patient than on a silicone mannequin. I held the paddles to Mr. Z's chest and simultaneously pressed the buttons on both paddles to send an electrical charge through his heart in hopes of resetting his heart's intrinsic pacemaker and restoring a normal rhythm. Just like that, Mr. Zimmerman's monitor showed a normal sinus rhythm indicating another successful cardioversion.

I was quietly pleased with myself. Jim had made it seem easy and comfortable, as though he could have handed the paddles to the janitor and gotten the same result. He probably could have. Most of all, Jim's confidence rubbed off on me, and confidence is also crucial to the practice of medicine. I felt like nothing bad would happen because Jim was right there, and if things went south, Jim would be there to fix it. He was, in no uncertain terms, "the man."

As we stood watch at the nursing station, my curiosity got the better of me. I asked Jim what had happened to Dr. Charlton's voice. Jim explained that Dr. Charlton had what was supposed to be relatively minor surgery but had sustained damage to his recurrent laryngeal nerve which affected his vocal cords.

I was feeling so great that I couldn't help but comment. "He sounds," I offered, "kind of like Marlon Brando in The Godfather." As soon as I heard myself say it, I winced at the thought that Jim might be less than thrilled that the FNG was making fun of one of the most revered professors in the entire department. Where was that little voice that I relied on?

Without missing a beat, Jim looked at me, tilting his head slightly to the side, and scratched his cheek with the backs of the tips of his fingers in a manner that I identified immediately. Then, in an impression that was dead-on, Jim uttered, "What have I ever done to make you treat me so disrespectfully?"

It was on.

Two grown men, devoted to healing the sick and comforting the dying, spent the rest of the evening in a reenactment of the entire Godfather trilogy, starring none other than cardiology guru Dr. Don Charlton.

Periodically, Mr. Zimmerman's cardiac monitor would signal an intermission, and we would once again zap his heart back into a normal rhythm.

Jim would then continue, "You come into my house on the day my daughter is to be married and you ask me to do a cardioversion, and for money. But you don't ask with respect. You don't offer friendship."

I chimed in, "If you had come to me in friendship then the vermin who ruined your heart rhythm would be suffering this very day."

I paused briefly, then looked at Jim and said, "I want you to arrange a meeting with the heads of the five services."

We spent the rest of the evening as the Godfathers, laughing until tears streamed down our faces. The nurses looked at us as though we were crazy. The fact is, we were. Some degree of insanity is prevalent in medicine. Well-honed defense mechanisms are necessary to see and treat mangled bodies without a second thought, or to tell a mother that her baby has just died.

While repeating movie line after movie line as only men do, our impersonations branched out to include other movies done by the cast of the Godfather, particularly Robert Duvall's character from Apocalypse Now, Lieutenant Colonel Bill Kilgore, who actually sounded a bit like the Godfather himself.

"Do you smell that?" Jim asked me. "Do you smell that? That's nitropaste, son. Nothing else in the world smells like that. I love the smell of nitropaste in the morning. You know one time we had a whole ward full of patients with angina, and after we laid nitropaste on all of them I walked up. We didn't find one of them, not one stinking patient with angina. But that smell, you know that nitropaste smell: the whole ward. Smelled like...victory."

I responded the only way I could, with a hint of melancholy in my voice: "Some day this rotation's going to end."

From that night on Dr. Charlton, esteemed cardiologist and researcher, was known simply as "the Don." As evening turned to late night and then to early morning, we grew tired and opted for trying to get some rest while there seemed to be lull in the action. As is always the case in medical training, though, just as the possibility of sleep arose, Mr. Zimmerman's alarm sounded once again. Jim lamented, "Just when I thought I was out, they pull me back in."

While that night was the first of many without sleep over the next five years, I'm glad I did it. I left the hospital around 6 p.m. the next day. Labor laws have since been enacted to prevent doctors and students from working such classic 36-hour shifts, but honestly, I never minded.

Toward the end of my cardiology rotation, I grew slightly bolder. One morning on rounds, I told Dr. Charlton that I thought my patient needed digoxin, a medication derived from the foxglove plant, which is used to treat arrhythmias and congestive heart failure.

"What dose do you want to give him?" he asked.

As almost all doctors tend to do early in their training, I low-balled it.

"0.125 milligrams every other day," I suggested.

He smirked, and prodded me, "Jesus, why don't you just wave the pill in front of his door? It would do him just as much good. Give him a manly dose. Try 0.25 milligrams a day."

Of course, I complied. Dr. Charlton understood my hesitance. Digoxin is a medication that can cause extremely dangerous side effects. It was completely normal for a physician in training to be reluctant to aggressively administer treatment with the potential to do more harm than good. After all, the purpose of medicine is to make people better, not worse. Accepting the fact that eventually you will harm a patient in an attempt to make them better is one of the more difficult realities of practicing medicine, but is critical to becoming an effective physician.

During rounds the next morning, Dr. Charlton again asked me about it, more to confirm that I had followed his orders than anything else.

"So, how much digoxin did you put him on?"

I was probably feeling bolder than I should have been when I responded.

"I didn't start him on digoxin."

He was puzzled, but somehow knew that there was no way a brand new third year medical student would simply ignore his orders. "Excuse me?"

"You said give him a manly dose. Real men don't take digoxin, Dr. Charlton. I gave him a foxglove plant and told him to chew on the leaves."

He laughed, then I quickly proceeded to tell him that I had followed his instructions to the letter and started the patient on 0.25 mg a day, more manly a dose than I had offered the day before, though perhaps not quite as macho as my alternative.

During my tenure on the cardiology service, I earned a Letter of Commendation. More importantly, I

learned three of the most important lessons in medicine from an intern named Jim: to separate the minutia from what is truly important; to, as Kipling once said, keep your head when all about you are losing theirs and blaming it on you; and perhaps most importantly, to practice medicine with a sense of humor.

CHAPTER TWO

Rounds

As a philosophy major, I admired the wisdom of Socrates and Plato. I was therefore excited when I was told that most of the direct teaching from attending physicians on clinical rotations was in the form of the Socratic method. "High level discussion among friends and colleagues," I assumed. Wrong!

This teaching occurred daily during "rounds." Rounds consisted of the entire medical team—medical students, interns, residents, fellows, and maybe a PharmD student—moving en masse with the attending physician from room to room as each patient on the ward was discussed and treatment plans developed and implemented.

I don't know what kind of sick perversion of the Socratic method rounds were supposed to emulate, but rounds were the scariest part of every day. For seemingly sadistic med school professors, rounds were an opportunity to excoriate and humiliate the pond scum of medical learning that we represented. The goal each and every day seemed to be to point out just what a dumbass I or one of my peers was, often in front of the patient. The funny thing was that I was accumulating well into six figures of debt to be treated in such a manner, so maybe I really *was* a dumbass!

My senior resident was, well, a douchebag. He was the epitome of a trust-fund frat-boy who drove his daddy's Bimmer with a "DR RIGHT" vanity plate. He attended Duke for medical school and managed to work that fact into almost every conversation, constantly belittling our medical school, which seemed odd since he was there for residency. I guess he couldn't get into internal medicine residency at Duke.

One day on rounds our attending noted an interesting physical exam finding in the patient's eyes: a linear pattern of small spots on the corneas of both eyes. He asked me what it was. I hadn't even noticed them, so of course I had no clue. He asked the other students. No idea. He asked the intern. Baffled. He finally asked our self-proclaimed genius of a senior resident, who also couldn't identify the physical exam finding.

"Maybe you could actually read a textbook and tell us all what it is tomorrow," the attending told me in front of the team.

"Yes, sir," I responded in crisp, clear military fashion.

That evening I studied physical exam findings of the eye in general and for nephrology patients specifically and discovered what I thought was the correct diagnosis. I was eager to check my answer with the attending the next morning.

The first rounds of the day consisted only of students, interns and residents to make sure we had our shit together before attending rounds. The resident asked me if I had looked up the answer. I told him I had.

"What is it?" he asked.

I responded, "It's called band keratopathy. Dialysis patients, who often have elevated calcium levels, can form calcium deposits on their corneas."

"Wrong!" he exclaimed with glee, as if he had just proven once again that I and the rest of my classmates never would have cut the mustard at Duke.

As a newbie, I simply assumed my diagnosis was incorrect and waited for him to tell me the correct answer.

"It's a pterygium," he declared.

I thought it odd, because I'd read about pterygium along with other eye findings and conditions the night before, and it didn't seem to fit the description to me. What did I know, though? This guy had four years of medical education on me. I had to assume he knew what he was talking about, even though he hadn't known the answer the day before, either, which meant he'd read about it just last night, same as me.

During attending rounds, we finally moved to the door in front of the patient's room. The attending hadn't forgotten the question. "So, Mr. Duling, what is the exam finding in this patient's eyes?"

The resident gave me a nod which seemed to half convey his pride that I would know the correct answer, and half reminding me that I shouldn't forget where I got it from.

"It's a pterygium," I said, undoubtedly sounding more like I had a question than an answer.

"No, Mr. Duling, it is not a pterygium," the attending said disappointedly. He didn't even bother giving me another shot. "Anyone else know the *correct* answer?" he inquired of the rest of the team.

No one said a word. I considered just taking my intellectual beating, which wasn't my first and wouldn't be my last, and slinking off to feel bad about myself when rounds were over. It was bugging me, though, to the point that I just spit out, "It's band keratopathy." I tried to sound more confident in this diagnosis. The attending seemed mildly surprised.

"Very good, Mr. Duling."

I made sure to glance directly at Mr. Duke.

The attending proceeded to ask me, "So, Mr. Duling, you probably noticed that this finding is only on the portion of the cornea that is exposed when his eyes are open. Why is that?"

"Wait. What? What kind of question was that?" I thought to myself. I'd studied all these eye findings the night before and figured out which one it was, unlike Mr. Duke. I even studied what caused it. I wasn't about to point it out to the attending, but in fact I had *not* noticed that it was only present on that portion of his eyes.

The attending explained in his typical, annoyed tone that band keratopathy formed on the interpalpebral portion of the cornea (which is doctor-speak for describing the part of the eye you can see when the eyes are open) because of the difference in pH resulting from lack of moisture and exposure to air.

That's how rounds went. If you knew the answer, good for you. There would always be one more question than you had answers. It pushed you to study all the answers you could find. It forced you to pay attention to detail. It made you a better doctor.

It was also uncomfortable as hell. Attending physicians were sharks, and med students were chum. It was a game you seemed to lose every day. Attending rounds always gave me that slightly nauseous feeling you get when you sit on the toilet in a public restroom and find the seat warm, but it was that discomfort that made you determined to raise your game a little more every day. Socrates knew what he was doing.

CHAPTER THREE

The First Time I Watched a Patient Die

Prior to medical school, I'd had only a few experiences with death. I vaguely recall the death of my great-grandmother on my mom's side. I remember seeing her in her apartment, using her walker, but don't really remember much else. On the evening that my parents dressed up to go to her wake, all I seemed to know was that something sad had happened.

The first death I truly remember was a classmate's in grade school.

Bonnie was the cutest girl in second grade. I was impressed with her from the start. She had short blonde bangs and a smile that made me want to chase her around the playground, as I seem to recall this was an appropriate first date for second grade. She had beautiful blue eyes, the kind you wanted to doodle with crayon. Bonnie was also the smartest kid in class. She was sweet, funny and kind as well—the whole package.

We played with Tinker Toys at my house or would swing outside at hers. As we lined up during a fire drill at school one day, I stood right behind her. Standing so close to her, I gathered the courage to tell her I liked her, and we hugged. I guess that meant we were an item, which translated to playing together almost every day.

Two years later, my fourth-grade teacher asked Bonnie and me to stay after class. Mrs. Dalton told us we were her two best students, that she had big expectations of us, and that she knew we would succeed in whatever we wanted to do in life. I was flabbergasted that Mrs. Dalton considered me to be in the same league as Bonnie. I was a good student, but Bonnie was exceptional. Mrs. Dalton was right, though. Bonnie could have achieved anything she wanted in life.

When fifth grade started, I was eager to renew my friendship with Bonnie. She lived at least ten blocks from my house, which at that age and time might as well have been ten states away, so I hadn't seen her all summer.

On the first day of school, Bonnie wasn't there. A mutual friend, Sheila, told me that Bonnie was sick. As the year passed, I rarely saw Bonnie. When I did, she looked different. Her face looked round but the rest of her was so skinny. Her hair looked wispy. As a ten-year-old, I had no idea what was wrong, but I knew something was.

One morning, while waiting with my classmates to climb the steps to class, Sheila spotted me from the top step, and she looked as though there was something she wanted to tell me, but the bell rang and she couldn't come back down the stairs as the herd began moving toward the door. We filed into the classroom, where she proceeded to tell me the shocking news. Bonnie, the smartest girl in my class with looks to match; the first girl I ever hugged; the girl who defined the traits I would seek in the woman I would marry, had died.

Bonnie's was the first funeral I ever attended. Her casket was open, and as I recall she looked like an angel. Her small hands clutched a bouquet of flowers. I reached up to touch the back of her hands and still remember their waxy feel. It just didn't seem real. Supposedly kids get a pretty good idea of death around the age of eight. I was ten. I'm not sure I understood. All I knew then was that a special little girl had died.

I've thought about Bonnie from time to time, especially since I became a doctor and a father. As an adult I learned that Bonnie had developed leukemia and had gone through chemotherapy. I then understood what happened to her hair, and realized that the round, swollen appearance of her face was probably induced by steroids, which cause the classic "moon facies" I was trained to recognize so many years later. At the age of ten I mourned Bonnie. As an adult I mourned for her parents and siblings.

Bonnie's was my first memorable experience with death. My next would hit closer to home.

My grandfather on my dad's side began to experience memory problems in his late 50's. I recall my dad and mom frantically running down the back porch and out into the street to track my grandfather down, as he had wandered off and they were afraid he was lost. As the years passed, he became more combative to the point that it was no longer safe for him to stay with my grandmother. Dementia robbed him of the ability to care for himself in any way, and he wound up in a nursing home.

My grandma cared for him devotedly. She fed him by spoon, washed him, combed his hair, and groomed him meticulously every time she visited him. Whenever I visited, his hands were wrapped in large mitts and tethered to the bed to keep him from scratching his skin off or taking a swing at the nursing staff. He didn't speak, and his room, for that matter the entire nursing home, always smelled strongly of urine.

I hated going there. I couldn't stand to see him like that. On Sundays, though, my family would drive Grandma to the nursing home and drop her off at the front door, then pick her up a few hours later. When I turned sixteen and got my driver's license, it became my responsibility to take her on Sundays. I never minded. At that age I was happy every time I got behind the wheel, and I would've done anything for my grandma. She was always special to me. She made the best chocolate chip cookies ever. She always told me I was her favorite grandson, which I just knew was the honest-to-goodness truth, despite the fact that I was her only grandson.

On the occasions I went into Grandpa's room at the nursing home to pick her up, I couldn't stand what I saw. He would moan incoherently and displayed no signs of recognition, even of his loyal wife. It was no way for a human being to live.

When my dad called my sister and me into the living room one Sunday morning, the little hairs on the back of my neck told me that it wasn't good. Grandpa had been very sick for a long time, and I inferred from my dad's tone that he had bad news to share with us. I had a feeling it was that Grandpa had died, and while I knew it was sad, I also breathed a sigh of relief, as death had to be better than his existence was. I was as prepared as I could be to hear the merciful, almost welcome news.

My dad's voice cracked slightly as he began to tell us. I could see he was upset, barely able to hold back his tears. I wanted to tell him not to fret.

"Really, Dad, it's OK. I'm glad he's not suffering anymore," I wanted to tell him.

He began to speak, "Your cousin Tracy was involved in a plane crash. She didn't survive. Tracy's dead."

It took a few moments for what he'd said to sink in.

"What? I thought Grandpa was dead?" I almost said aloud. This couldn't be true. He misspoke. How the hell would he mix up Grandpa with Tracy?

He saw that we weren't processing the information, and he understood why, so he repeated it. As I began to comprehend what had happened, I was devastated.

Tracy was wickedly funny. She was the type of person who would light up a room and put everyone at ease. She always made it a point to come see us, even when she was home from college, as she was just nineteen at the time of her death.

My aunt and uncle asked me to be a pall bearer, which I considered an honor. They knew that I had always looked up to her. After the funeral, as the family gathered at their church for some food and condolences, sharing memories of a life taken far too soon, I wandered out back and sat on the back step. My uncle came out and sat down next to me. I started to cry. He consoled me. I guess it's what you would expect an adult to do with a teenager, but decades later, I marvel at the strength it must have taken. He had lost his youngest of three daughters, yet *he* had the strength to console *me*.

My grandfather, who I had expected to hear had died that Sunday morning, actually died a year later, another year of living in a state none of us would wish on our worst enemies. My sorrow began to transform to anger. He developed pneumonia over the winter, and I thought surely that would bring the long-awaited merciful end. He was "treated successfully," however, and lived another eight months before succumbing. He'd spent seven horrific years in that nursing home, the last four of which he spent tied to his bed, completely unaware of his surroundings and unable to communicate with anyone about anything. This fourth experience tempered my understanding of death as a terrible loss with the realization that death wasn't always the worst thing that could happen to a person.

I had been quite fortunate that these were the only four experiences with death I'd had upon entering medicine. We all bring into the profession our biases, prejudices, religious beliefs (or, in my case, lack thereof), and an approach to death based on our values. A physician's outlook on death can profoundly influence how a patient or a patient's family reacts when difficult decisions have to be made. I wanted to be an ER doc more than anything; to save lives; to be the hero who swoops in and snatches the patient back from the brink of death, giving them more time to hug and make memories with their loved ones. Watching my grandfather suffer and wither away, however, made me realize for the first time that maybe there are some fates worse than death. How would I know the difference? How would I learn when to fight by any means necessary and when to submit, allowing a peaceful death and maintaining the patient's dignity? This question is what drove me to study philosophy and medical ethics rather than biochemistry or molecular biology. I wasn't going to be a scientist. I was going to save lives in all manner of ways on the front lines in the ER.

My first experience with death during medical school was a different type of encounter altogether, one that started on my very first day.

Gross Anatomy is the cornerstone of a medical education. All other medical learning builds on and stems from knowledge of what's where in the human body. The way you learned this was by dissecting a human cadaver. We were assigned four students per cadaver and spent the first thirteen weeks of medical school completely devoted to learning the anatomy of the human body.

I stared at the body, which smelled strongly of formaldehyde, but immediately before the first cut was made, I had a strange sense. A chill went down my spine and it was almost as if an absolute truth had been revealed to me in those few moments. As I examined this preserved body, I had an existential moment, wondering what it was that gave us this thing we call life. Was it really simply an infinite series of complex biological processes, or was there was some intangible quality that made us human beings? Was there such thing as a soul, some kind of magic that took these parts—these molecules, cells, tissues and organs—and made them into... us? I still don't pretend to know.

I had other experiences with death in medical school, of course. For the most part, though, hearing "Code Blue, Room 842, Code Blue, Room 842, Code Blue, Room 842" overhead meant you better run if you wanted to get in on the action. In a large teaching hospital, if you weren't on the same floor, or maybe one floor above or below but right next to the stairway closest to the patient's room, forget about it; by the time you got there, a crowd of fifty white coats had gathered, and you wouldn't even be able to see inside the room. As a medical student, if you were lucky enough to get inside the room, your only job was to perform chest compressions. This was fascinating enough by itself, but watching the interns and residents intubate, medicate, and defibrillate the patient was awe-inspiring.

During my trauma surgery rotation as a third-year medical student, I saw my first traumatic death of a young person, as opposed to the death of an elderly person from illness. A nineteen-year-old boy had been drinking and ran his car into a tree. He was essentially DOA (dead on arrival), and after a brief, unsuccessful attempt at resuscitation, he was quickly pronounced dead. His injuries were obvious and multiple. As a student trying to accurately document his injuries, not to mention absorb the sight of one of the first mangled bodies I had seen, I lingered in the room after the rest of the trauma team had left except for one nurse. The ER nurse was using a warm, wet washcloth to wipe the blood off his face and torso, trying to somehow make him look presentable to his family when they came to see him. Then she said something that has stuck with me ever since.

"Look what you have done to your mother tonight."

In that instant, the reality of the situation struck me as if it were lightning. I felt like sobbing for the first time in my medical career. It wasn't the last. I was glad my back was turned to the nurse. At the time, I thought it would appear weak to cry in front of her.

I'd had a couple of other brushes with death to that point in life. As a medic in the Army, I was able to witness an autopsy on a 7-year-old girl who had become ill one night. She climbed into bed between her parents because she wasn't feeling well, and when they woke up in the morning, she lay dead between them. After peeling back her scalp and cutting the top of her skull off, the pathologist showed me what meningitis looked like, clouding what should have been a clear covering of the brain.

While in medical school, I responded to the sound of a neighbor shrieking after discovering her aged father dead in his favorite chair. Even as a first-year medical student, I could recognize rigor mortis and the lack of need for any attempt at resuscitation.

These experiences were important to me. They were meaningful. The most profound experience with death I would have as a medical student was yet to come, though.

In the winter of my fourth year, I was doing a rotation in the SICU (Surgical Intensive Care Unit). It was a tough but rewarding month, as the SICU was filled with incredibly sick patients, including several transplant patients. One Friday morning, one of my classmates announced to the team that he had a family wedding to attend that weekend, and therefore split his patients up among the rest of us. We each assumed responsibility for them accordingly. He told me about Sebastian, a patient who had been in the SICU for a week now. I had heard

Sebastian's story on morning rounds every day that week. It was tragic.

Sebastian was a 32-year-old juvenile-onset diabetic. Insulin-dependent diabetes is a terrible disease to have as a child and young adult. Managing it safely requires giving yourself repeated daily injections of insulin and poking your finger several times a day to check your blood sugar. You have to watch what you eat very closely, which is particularly difficult for teenagers, who want nothing more than to go out with their friends and grab a pizza. At the time, if you were diagnosed early in life, by the time you were in your late twenties you probably already had serious complications of your disease. Diabetes causes retinopathy (which leads to blindness), nephropathy (kidney failure, which leads to dialysis), neuropathy (which destroys nerves and can result in weakness or constant, searing pain), vasculopathy (blood vessel problems which can lead to amputations, heart attacks, and strokes), and multiple other problems including severe infections. Type I, or "juvenile-onset," diabetes is caused by a failure of your pancreas to produce insulin.

Sebastian had been a type I diabetic for over twenty years, and his kidneys had failed. He had been on dialysis, which is never an appealing option at any age, let alone as a young man. His best option was to receive a kidney-pancreas transplant. The transplant, if successful, could dramatically improve his quality of life. No more pokes. No more insulin. No more watching every carbohydrate. Certainly, there were significant risks of being a transplant patient, namely the potent anti-rejection medications one had to take which predisposed you to nasty infections. If all went well, though, and barring rejection, a kidney-pancreas transplant gave Sebastian a good chance at a much more normal life for a young man.

Sebastian had received his kidney-pancreas transplant earlier that week and initially seemed to be doing well post-operatively. Abruptly, for no apparent reason, he went into cardiac arrest. He was still intubated from surgery, and CPR was initiated. He was given three rounds of medications, epinephrine and atropine, and his heart finally restarted. By the time it had, however, the damage was done. Since his cardiac arrest, Sebastian hadn't responded. He wasn't brain-dead, but both the transplant and ICU teams had been following him closely, and he showed no signs of improvement. Discussions had been initiated about potentially withdrawing support.

We had all avoided going into that room all week. It was almost as if you tuned the whole thing out if he wasn't your patient. The rest of us who were not directly involved in his care didn't need to know about such terrible things. You had enough of them to worry about with your own patients without getting emotionally involved with someone else's. On that Friday, though, I wouldn't have a choice. He would be my patient for the weekend.

I took a deep breath and entered the room to find Sebastian surrounded by IV poles and pumps that were administering what must have been ten different medications through his veins in a valiant attempt to save his life. His young wife stood beside him, holding his hand. His father sat in a chair next to the bed. Apparently, there was a large contingent of family and friends with him, but most of them had gone to get something to eat. The hospital tried to limit the number of visitors in a patient's room at one time. Exceptions were generally made for the dying, however.

As I spoke to his wife, she indicated that many of them had traveled a long way to get there, as she and Sebastian were not from Columbus.

"Where are you from?" I asked, trying to generate any small talk I could think of.

"Toledo," she responded.

"No kidding, I'm from Toledo." I told her.

"Really? What part?"

"I'm from West Toledo."

"So am I," she said. I was thankful that we had something to chat about other than her dying husband.

"Where did you go to high school?" she asked.

"Roosevelt."

She paused briefly.

"What year did you graduate?" she inquired.

"1984," I told her.

She paused again, looked at my face for some type of recognition, then she floored me.

"Me too."

"What?" I asked incredulously.

"I graduated from Roosevelt in '84."

I asked her maiden name, and though the name sounded familiar, I searched my memory banks for any recollection of her, but it was clear that we hadn't known each other. Our graduating class had almost eight hundred students, and each of our social circles were considerably smaller than that. Still, we were both amazed that of all the odd things that could have happened on that day, two former high school classmates met for the first time almost eleven years after graduation, one nearly a doctor and the other nearly a widow.

I instantly felt more comfortable, though the side effect was that I also felt an instant connection. We chatted about all that had happened, and about how much she loved Sebastian and what a great guy he was. His father seemed glad to know that someone would be looking after him who had this connection to the family, no matter how remote.

It was evident that day, however, that Sebastian had reached the end of the line. There was nothing more that could be done for him. He was going to die. I stood silently behind the senior members of the team on rounds as the attending physician explained to Sebastian's wife and family that the time had come to let him go. He was receiving multiple forms of "life support": his breathing was controlled by the ventilator, and he was on numerous drips to support his heart rate, blood pressure, the function of his new kidney, and to fight off any infections. Those who loved and cared for Sebastian made the only decision they knew they could: turn everything off and let him go peacefully.

That afternoon, all the pumps and medications were removed except for some saline (saltwater) just to keep some fluids in him. The ventilator was turned off and he was extubated. It was thought that with the level of support he was receiving to keep him alive, it wouldn't be long before he succumbed after a long, courageous fight. As often happens in these instances, though, it didn't turn out that way. Sebastian's chest heaved as he took a gasp just often enough to keep going. His heart rate didn't change much. Neither did his blood pressure.

I spent the day popping into Sebastian's room frequently to check on him, more so to check on his wife and the rest of his family and friends. We had several conversations about Sebastian, about Toledo, about high school, and about what would happen next.

Afternoon turned to evening, then to night. Sebastian continued to cling to life. Everyone was exhausted. Nobody knew how long the process might take. At about midnight the family decided to go back to their hotels. I was on call that night and assured them that I would call them if anything happened.

Before she left, Sebastian's wife looked at me with tears in her eyes and asked, "Please don't leave him alone. I don't want him to be alone."

I told her I would stay with him all night. Normally when you're on call you try to sleep every chance you get, but on this night, sleep didn't mean anything. I'd gone without sleep many times before: what was one more night? It was my duty to stay with Sebastian.

The rest of the unit was eerily quiet. I got a chill when I realized what I was about to do. I had seen dead people before, but I had never seen someone actually die- to just sit and watch the life drain slowly from what not so long ago was a robust, walking, talking, thinking, laughing human being. I wanted to cry but felt like I couldn't. This was an important part of becoming a doctor, right? How could I be a doctor without seeing death up close, watching it, studying it?

Death is the enemy of medicine. At least that's the way we've always treated it. Death is an enemy to be fought at all costs. Surrender is not in our creed, and defeat is never accepted or taken lightly. Some may think it sounds noble. Some may think we're playing God. Both views are somewhat valid. Our job is to interfere with nature in an attempt to improve the quality and quantity of patients' lives. I was devoting my life to fighting death. Death *is* the enemy. But as I knew from my experiences with my grandfather, sometimes there are worse things than dying. Part of the problem in medicine, and in society, is that we often don't know when to surrender to it, when to stop fighting it; when, as Dylan Thomas phrased it, to go gently into that good night.

I watched Sebastian do it. I sat at the foot of his bed for two hours. His pulse began to slow, as did his breathing. He began to gasp in an irregular pattern that indicated the end was near. His heart rate slowed from over 100 earlier in the day to the 50's, then 40's, then 30's. His body was slowing down and would soon be stopped forever. Whatever mystical life force makes us what and who we are was leaving Sebastian. It was a powerful thing to witness.

His heart rhythm became agonal as the monitor showed a blip only once every several seconds now. He gasped once more, seemed almost to hold it for a few seconds, and then released it slowly. That breath was his last. As the last bit of air flowed out, Sebastian smiled.

I did a double take. Had I actually just seen that? He *smiled*?! Had he seen something on the other side that put him at ease and allowed him to smile again? None of us will ever know until we're there ourselves.

I sat for a few moments, trying to absorb all that I had just seen. It was important to remember. Somehow it would make me a better doctor. I didn't want to forget. I haven't.

I picked up the phone and called his wife. She knew what it meant when the phone rang. I've always believed that when someone dies in a hospital, a doctor should be the one to tell the family. It is a solemn responsibility that should not be dished off on a nurse, chaplain, or student. A human being has died in the hospital. The family deserves to hear from a physician when the life of a loved one has ended. In this case, however, I felt I was the best person to tell her, though I was still a few months short of being a doctor.

I've found that you never know how a death will affect you. I hope I never reach the point when death doesn't affect me. If I do, it's probably time to do something else.

CHAPTER FOUR

Why I Became an ER Doc

I told you that my cousin died in a plane crash. The part I didn't tell you was that she survived the impact of the crash but was severely injured and was burned over 90% of her body. She was so disfigured and unrecognizable that another surviving passenger confused her with the other girl on board. As the crash occurred on a remote mountain on an island in the Caribbean, it took almost 24 hours for the rescue crew to locate and arrive at the crash scene. She reportedly lived for most of that time, dying shortly before help arrived.

When her remains were returned to Michigan, she had to be identified by family. My aunt and uncle were very kind and loving people. Family meant everything to them. My dad didn't think her mother or father should be the ones to see her body first, so he went in their place. After confirming it was her, my father convinced his sister and brother-in-law that they shouldn't see her like that. He knew the image would stick with them always, and he believed no parent should spend the rest of their days with that memory.

Even as a teenager, I was in awe of that. It was such an act of kindness, of love, of mercy. It took such strength. My dad was the rock of our family. He never seemed rattled. He was always the go-to guy. Everyone could depend on him for anything. I didn't realize until many years later that it took an incredible toll on my dad as well.

I've told my kids that story about Grandpa. When I was 53 and my parents, 78 years of age at the time, were visiting us, my son mentioned it, and my dad started crying. I had never said anything to him about it—that I knew what he'd done, that I'd thought about it from time to time over the years, or that it helped shape me as a person. After almost 40 years, it still haunted him, though I think he was also reacting to knowing that his son and grandkids knew what he'd done and, perhaps for the first time, that someone else understood.

Like most boys, I wanted to emulate the best of my dad. I wanted to be strong. I wanted to be someone people could depend on and lean on. I wanted to be the one to do the hard things at the most difficult times. I wanted to be someone people could turn to in a crisis.

Also typical of young males, I liked shiny red ambulances. Growing up in Toledo, the ambulances had "REMSNO" on their sides: Regional Emergency Medical Services of Northwest Ohio. When I saw one with lights and sirens racing off somewhere, I wondered where they were going, and who had to deal with it on the other end. When I heard the Life Flight helicopter overhead, I looked to the sky with curiosity. Where would the chopper land, and who was waiting for it when it did?

I took a first aid course for a semester in high school and loved it. I had always thought about a career in medicine, in no small part because my dad thought it was the best thing a smart person could be. When my parents discovered I was a relatively sharp kid, even if I wasn't always a great student, they'd constantly say, "You should be a doctor or a lawyer." At one point I remember saying, "Being a lawyer would be cool," to which my dad would sound annoyed and say, "There are a lot more starving lawyers than there are starving doctors!" While I'm pretty sure they would have been proud had I gone to law school, it was clear which profession was preferred.

I enlisted into the U.S. Army when I was 17 under the Delayed Entry Program, meaning I finished my senior year of high school and went to boot camp that summer, after I'd turned 18. I had a strong sense of patriotism and wanted to serve my country. I joined as a 91A, a "Combat Medical Specialist." It was 1984, near the end of Ronald Reagan's first term, back when we all acknowledged that Russia was our enemy. The Cold War remained frigid and tensions were high as we continued to resist their efforts to undermine democracy around the world.

I figured being a medic in the Army would let me serve my country while gaining valuable experience and insight to the medical field, just to make sure I liked it before investing all the time and effort into a career in medicine.

After almost four years on Active Duty as a medic, I found the medical field to be so unbelievably boring that there was no way I could see myself doing that for a career. My experiences were limited to working as an orderly during a three-month rotation in a hospital, pulling sick call in our Battalion Aid Station, and a rotation at the local dispensary, which was like an Urgent Care. To put it plainly, I thought medicine was a snooze-fest. While I still thought the art of healing was noble, it definitely was not for me.

I therefore decided to pursue what I was most passionate about at the time. I planned to study electrical engineering, determined to design hi-fi stereo equipment like Dr. Bose at M.I.T, Matthew Polk, or Bob Carver. After four years in the Army, however, I had some catching up to do. One year into college, I realized that it would take me five years to successfully complete a B.S.

in Electrical Engineering. I became restless and reevaluated my life goals.

I found myself drifting back to medicine. In the intervening years since my adolescence, I'd learned where all those ambulances and helicopters went with the most critical patients. They went to the emergency room, where they were seen by ER doctors. "How cool must that job be?" I pondered.

I switched majors, first to biology, because every pre-med student seemed to be either a biology or a chemistry major. Not particularly caring for either one, I chose what I thought was the lesser of two evils. At the same time, I began researching what I needed to do in order to get into medical school. The guidebook I purchased indicated that you could study anything you wanted, so long as you completed the prerequisites: one year each of calculus, biology, chemistry, physics and organic chemistry. Other than those math and science requirements, my college degree could be in anything I wanted to study.

Recalling my grandfather's last years in a nursing home and my innate sense that it was immoral to let a human being die that way, I became enthralled with medical ethics. I was determined to fight the injustice of forcing patients to live horrible, demeaning existences before letting them die from suffocation due to pneumonia, languishing away until their skin and bones could no longer sustain life, or any number of other intolerable and undignified endings. I felt strongly that the tools that would best prepare me for a career in medicine included a comprehensive study of medical ethics.

I also did the math. By changing majors again, I could be halfway through medical school by the time I would have obtained a BSEE. That's just what I did, obtaining a B.A. in Philosophy in three years at the University of Toledo, my hometown school and, frankly, the only college I could afford to attend. I completed my Honors Thesis in medical ethics. After applying to medical school at The Ohio State University, I was fortunate enough to have an interview with a PhD who was in charge of the Medical Humanities Program. To this day, I remain convinced that my somewhat unusual background, being a 25-year-old veteran with a degree in philosophy (and, to be fair, pretty good MCAT scores) was the primary reason I was accepted.

I was even more thrilled to start medical school when I learned that Ohio State would be offering a brand-new curriculum, an experimental program called Problem-Based Learning, or PBL. Rather than sitting in lecture halls several hours a day Monday through Friday, we would meet three times a week for two hours each, and the rest of our learning would be independent study.

Each small group session consisted of six students and two faculty members. A case was presented on paper as a real patient might present, usually in the emergency department. I still recall the first case, a fictional yet realistic patient named Agatha Willis. Despite the fact that we spent the first thirteen weeks of medical school completing an intensive course in Gross Anatomy, the cleverness of the patient's name was lost on me as we were told her chief complaint: severe headache.

The case unfolded over a few sessions. We had no idea where to start. We knew nothing about taking a history or performing a physical examination. We'd never interpreted a lab result, looked at an x-ray or prescribed a medication. The point of the first two years of medical school is to learn the "basic sciences," the scientific knowledge and principles that form the foundation of the rest of one's medical education. These disciplines included anatomy, physiology, biochemistry, histology, embryology, microbiology, pharmacology and pathophysiology. The endpoint was taking Part I of the USMLE (United

States Medical Licensing Exam), a three-part series of exams taken after the second year of medical school, near the end of the fourth year of medical school, and after completing an internship. Passing all three parts meant you were a full-fledged doctor. Doctors generally go on to complete residencies in their chosen fields, mine being emergency medicine, but technically you could hang out a shingle and call yourself a "GP" (General Practitioner) after passing all three phases of the USMLE.

As we explored the case of Agatha Willis, we identified "learning issues," things we needed to study to develop an understanding of her presentation, and to be able to diagnose and treat her properly, at least on paper. Given that we had just started week 14 of medical school, it was hard to narrow the topics down, but we were guided by faculty to choose some and dove into studying them. We decided to learn about types of headaches and the typical presentations of each, as well as some neurology, tips on taking a history, and some pharmacology.

The cleverness I mentioned referred to her diagnosis. Agatha had a ruptured cerebral aneurysm, something that most commonly occurs in the confluence of arteries in your head called the Circle of Willis. Agatha Willis. If only every patient presented with such a clue in their name, emergency medicine would be a whole lot easier.

We studied case after case, and the learning issues piled up. The theory behind problem-based learning was that it should better prepare you for your clinical years of medical training starting in your third year, when you actually went into the hospital and started seeing real patients and learning how medicine is practiced in real time.

There was a healthy amount of skepticism about the potential for problem-based learning in a medical school environment, but the enthusiasm for the program by its founder at Ohio State, Dr. John Curry, PhD, was contagious among us PBL students. I am biased, certainly, but our first class of PBL students was highly motivated to jump into an experimental program, and we were comfortable with the notion of taking our education into our own hands. Dr. Curry inspired trust and confidence that he wouldn't steer us wrong. He didn't. The goal of the first two years of medical school was to prepare you for Part I of the boards; our first PBL class earned higher average test scores than the lecture students.

Throughout the first two years of medical school, I didn't lose sight of my passion for medical ethics. I created a brown-bag lunch series focused on hot-button issues of the day in medical ethics. During this time, the most public and controversial medical ethics issue was driven by a previously unknown pathologist from Royal Oak, Michigan named Dr. Jack Kevorkian.

Dr. Kevorkian sparked a national debate about physician-assisted suicide, going to prison multiple times to fight for what he saw as a fundamental human right guaranteed to us in the Constitution. I happened to agree wholeheartedly.

While I was fiercely passionate about end-of-life issues, however, what I wanted to do more than anything was to save lives in the ER. Most students start medical school because they know they want to be doctors, then they figure out which specialty they want to practice during their journey through med school. Not me. I knew exactly what kind of doctor I wanted to be. I went to medical school to become an ER doc.

During each rotation, I paid particular attention to the skills and knowledge I would need to practice emergency medicine and, honestly, had little time or patience for anything irrelevant to my chosen profession.

I loved every minute of emergency medicine residency. The hours were long, the work exhausting, but the reward was the sense of accomplishment and confidence in one's ability to serve others. Some lessons were easily learned, others the hard way. Those were magical years in my life; I didn't want to be anywhere else. There's a saying in medicine: "The only problem with every other night call is that you miss so much on your night off."

During one of my trauma surgery rotations, I once spent 145 of the possible 168 hours that constitute a week in the hospital. Was that absolutely ridiculous and probably uncalled for? Sure. But it also instilled in me a sense of accomplishment. It felt like I belonged. It is probably pathological, because that's why doctors begin to feel they are superhuman, unencumbered by the physical and mental limits of mortals. We aren't, of course, and we, our patients and society at large would be much better off if we all recognized the human failings of doctors and extended understanding and compassion to them.

There is no place I'd rather be in the house of medicine than in the ER. There are no finer people with whom I could possibly work. I chose to be where smart people were needed when the shit hit the fan. It is a humbling responsibility, to be sure, but that's why I became an ER doctor.

CHAPTER FIVE

Back From the Dead

While death is an inescapable part of the medical profession, we don't spend years studying and training just to watch someone die; we want to save lives. There are different ways to do that in medicine. The best way is to prevent people from becoming ill. Physicians can encourage patients to exercise, eat a healthy diet, lose weight, stop smoking, avoid drinking to excess, perform screening medical exams like mammograms and colonoscopies, wear seat belts and helmets, properly secure firearms, child-proof their homes, get vaccinations, and generally make smart, science-based decisions to lead longer, healthier and happier lives. Preventive medicine is perhaps the most important and effective type of medical intervention.

Doctors also help save lives by treating diseases in order to avoid serious complications, such as by managing hypertension over decades to prevent a stroke or heart attack, or treating diabetes to prevent kidney failure, blindness or amputations.

In more acute disease, doctors intervene more urgently to prevent dire consequences. Examples include appendectomies and antibiotic therapy for pneumonia. Left untreated, these disease processes could lead to permanent disability or death.

Emergent intervention to prevent imminent death is the stuff of legend. An obstetrician performs an emergent cesarean delivery of a fetus with an umbilical cord around its neck whose heart rate becomes dangerously slow. An interventional cardiologist opens a coronary artery to reestablish blood flow to heart muscle during a heart attack. An interventional neuroradiologist retrieves a blood clot that causes a stroke. A neurosurgeon drills a hole in a skull to remove a blood clot causing increased pressure on the brain.

One of most intense and rewarding experiences in emergency medicine, however, isn't preventing death or even stopping death in its tracks as it is occurring. It's reversing death—snatching a patient from the jaws of death back into the land of the living.

It doesn't happen very often. Dead people tend to stay that way.

Before we proceed, you need to understand how death is defined. We all have a pretty clear concept of death, right? The details are not always as clear as you might think, however. See if you can answer these two questions:

- Explain how a patient with a strong pulse and normal blood pressure can be dead.
- Explain how a patient with no pulse can be alive.

If you know the answers, chances are pretty good that you either work in the medical field or have tragic personal experience with these concepts.

Let's start with the latter: how can a person with no pulse be alive? Answer: the patient has a Left Ventricular Assist Device, or LVAD. It's basically a heart pump. An impeller in the pump spins thousands of RPM, putting out continuous blood flow, yet the patient has no pulse. Normally, when our heart contracts, it pumps blood forward with each heartbeat, and we feel each surge in pressure as our pulse. An LVAD keeps the blood constantly flowing with no "surges" that we can feel as a pulse. Fascinating, isn't it?

Now, how can a patient with a strong pulse and normal blood pressure be dead? This is more complicated. We define death in two ways: clinical death and biological death.

Clinical death means your heart has stopped and you aren't breathing. Once you are clinically dead, the rest of you isn't getting any oxygen delivery; the organ most sensitive to this is your brain. Within 4–6 minutes without oxygen and blood flow, brain cells start to die. This is known as biological death, which is irreversible. Once cells are dead, they're permanently dead. It's not as if every brain cell dies by exactly six minutes, however, which is why some people who suffer a cardiac arrest and have a prolonged "down time" survive. The more time goes by and the more brain cells lost to lack of oxygen and blood flow, the higher the odds of getting a heartbeat back only to lose vital cognitive functions, which is how people end up in a persistent vegetative state, living "like a vegetable," a fate we should all want to avoid.

Once your brain has been denied oxygen long enough, you are brain dead. Your heart might continue beating. This scenario occurs with some regularity, and is how young, otherwise healthy people become organ donors. A 21-year-old riding a motorcycle without a helmet crashes and smacks his head into a guard rail. His brain swells from the blunt trauma, cutting off blood flow and oxygen supply to his brain; he is brain dead. He's not going to recover. He's not coming back. Ever.

Yet our brain-dead 21-year-old trauma patient has a heart that is, well, the heart of a healthy 21-year-old, meaning it might beat for another 70 years. The same is true for his kidneys, lungs, liver, pancreas and other organs and tissues that can be "harvested" (that term has never sounded right to me) and used to save the lives of numerous people on transplant waiting lists across the country. A brain-dead patient can have a strong pulse and normal blood pressure yet can be declared legally dead.

How often are we successful at bringing patients back from clinical death? Not very often. Almost 350,000 people experience OHCA (Out of Hospital Cardiac Arrest) each year. 90% of them do not survive to hospital discharge. It is important to understand the relevance of that metric. EMS agencies and emergency departments do an amazing job in doing everything they can to save people in the event of cardiac arrest. During a "Code" (resuscitation), the best words you can hear are "We've got a pulse." This indicates a ROSC, return of spontaneous circulation, meaning the patient has a heartbeat again.

Unfortunately, this is often temporary, as whatever process caused the patient to die in the first place can't be fixed, or the damage done is too great, and the patient dies sometime later. Only 10% live long enough to be discharged from the hospital, and only 8% survive relatively intact. In other words, even if you are fortunate enough to survive a cardiac arrest, you may never be the same.

Which is why, on the few occasions in your career when you are able to bring a patient back from being clinically dead to walking out the door to spend more time with their families and loved ones, it ranks among the most exhilarating, rewarding and emotional experiences an ER doctor, or any health care provider for that matter, can experience.

Your odds of successfully bringing someone back from the dead depend on what caused clinical death in the first place. If someone sees you drop dead and immediately does CPR or grabs an AED (automated external defibrillator) and shocks your heart back into a normal rhythm, your odds are much better than if you dropped dead from a ruptured abdominal aortic aneurysm.

One of the most common clinical-death scenarios currently encountered by ER physicians is the patient in respiratory arrest from opioid overdose. Given the national crisis of opioid-related deaths, this occurs far too frequently. The treatment is fairly straightforward; naloxone (Narcan) is administered. You can give it intravenously, squirt it down an endotracheal tube if the patient has already been intubated, or most commonly these days, give it intra-nasally. The nasal spray is the fastest, easiest way to administer it.

While these scenarios make for a pretty exciting shift in the ER, there remains a category of patients who are clinically dead but for whom standard resuscitation measures like naloxone, CPR or defibrillation would never work, for whom their only chance at life is to have a doctor quickly figure out what's wrong with them and know how to fix it immediately.

One such case occurred when I responded to a Code Blue in the ICU. The patient had just lost her pulse and was already on a ventilator. CPR had been initiated. She was in PEA, pulseless electrical activity, which means that the monitor showed what looked like a good heart rhythm, but there was no pulse to go with it. As luck would have it, a chest x-ray had just been taken shortly before the patient arrested, and the x-ray tech brought the film up as CPR was in progress. This was back in the days of old-fashioned x-ray films, when you had to put the film up on a lightbox to interpret it. I held the x-ray up to the light with one hand while the index and middle fingers of my other hand remained anchored over her femoral artery as chest compressions were administered. I identified a "pleural line" with nothing but air peripheral to it, meaning that one of her lungs was completely collapsed. She had a tension pneumothorax. There was a leak in her lung, and air was escaping from the lung into the chest cavity around it, ultimately building up enough pressure that it not only collapsed her lung but also prevented blood from returning to her heart, resulting in the loss of her pulse.

Despite the fact that I was in an intensive care unit, no one could locate a needle large enough to penetrate her chest wall to release the pressure in her chest, nor could anyone find a chest tube kit. Since she was quite thin, I asked for a 10-blade (a scalpel) and made an incision in her left lateral chest wall. Not having instruments or time for someone to look for any, I used my finger to tunnel up the soft tissues along her rib cage and was able to poke my finger between her ribs and into her chest cavity. I felt and heard a large rush of air indicating that I had decompressed the tension pneumothorax. Within a few seconds her pulse returned. It worked—she was alive!

Unfortunately, while I won the battle, the war was destined to be lost. The patient was intubated in the ICU for a reason. She was at the end of a long battle with cancer and died in the hospital two days later. She never woke up, never spoke to her family again. In the end, all I did was delay the inevitable by a couple of days.

Even in a hospital, the best place you could possibly be if your heart stops, only 20% of patients who experience cardiac arrest survive. No matter how heroic every nurse and doctor want to be, we don't control the outcome.

Three times in my career, though, a patient has been brought to my ER by ambulance in cardiac arrest with CPR in progress due to one specific diagnosis yet lived to tell about it. It sounds like a precise number, but consider the context. We're not talking about the patient who drops dead from a heart attack, gets defibrillated and comes back to life. Bringing a patient back from the dead that way will always be one of the most amazing experiences an ER team can share.

I'm talking about three patients who couldn't just be shocked back to life; they required a rapid, accurate diagnosis just in the nick of time to save their lives.

I'll give you two hints. For one patient, the medics described her rhythm as "like a slow V-tach," meaning a wide-complex QRS complex with a slow rate. For another, the medics said she went into cardiac arrest after showing up for her dialysis appointment.

For an emergency physician, each of those is a pretty strong clue pointing to one thing: hyperkalemia, or high potassium. While some patients may experience symptoms as their potassium climbs, it is not unusual for the patient to feel nothing until their heart stops from a fatal level of potassium.

What do the clues mean? Well, dialysis is the easier one. Excess potassium is excreted through your kidneys. If your kidneys don't work, you can't get rid of potassium, and the only way to keep your potassium at a safe level is through routine dialysis, usually three days a week, on say Mon-Wed-Fri or Tue-Thu-Sat. As soon as you complete a dialysis treatment, you have few other mechanisms to regulate your acid-base balance, eliminate excess fluid from your body, or lower your potassium. The fact that my patient had just showed up for dialysis was a strong clue that she likely had a buildup of fluid, acid and/or potassium in her blood, and hyperkalemia was the one most likely to result in sudden cardiac arrest.

My patient with "slow V-tach" triggered my recollection of an axiom of medicine: *wide and fast is V-tach until proven otherwise, wide and slow is hyperkalemia until proven otherwise*. Admittedly, this is getting into the weeds; let me just say that doctors spend a lot of time mastering basic sciences to understand the action potential, ion channels, depolarization and repolarization, the cardiac cycle, and so on and so on, as well as the effect that too much potassium has on these biological processes. It adds up to being able to immediately recognize that when a medic describes the patient's heart rhythm on the monitor as deteriorating from something that looked fairly normal to something that was now wide and slow, followed by cardiac arrest, that is precisely the evolution of changes one might see as hyperkalemia worsens to become fatal.

When I explain hyperkalemia to patients, I tend to use the following illustration of just how dangerous hyperkalemia is. Admittedly, it sometimes freaks them out, but I want to instill a bit of fear and relay the deadly serious nature of hyperkalemia to them. As such, I explain that high potassium is so effective at stopping the heart that "we," the people of the United States, use it to execute people.

That's right—when states routinely used a three-drug cocktail to execute death row prisoners, the first drug was usually a short-acting barbiturate. This was administered in a dose sufficient to kill people by itself, as it induced a state of general anesthesia and would stop most people from breathing. The second drug was a paralytic agent, which paralyzed the muscles that make us breathe, without which we suffocate and die. Given the massive dose of sedative already on board, we'd never feel it, though.

The third and final drug, the coup de grâce, was potassium. Potassium is a cardioplegic drug. You're familiar with the terms "paraplegic" or "quadriplegic", when two or four limbs are paralyzed, or don't move. Cardio-plegic means heart-doesn't move. Heart not moving = bad.

A less macabre example of the use of potassium as a cardioplegic agent is in open heart surgery. If you need bypass surgery, the anesthesiologist and heart surgeons will place you on a bypass pump, then potassium will be administered to stop your heart while they work on it. Pretty amazing.

Life-threatening hyperkalemia is managed emergently by first administering calcium intravenously followed by sodium bicarbonate, insulin (with or without glucose), and nebulized albuterol. These treatments don't actually get rid of extra potassium; they shift the potassium in your body around long enough to restore a functional heart rhythm. Dialysis is then performed emergently to remove the excess potassium from your body.

All three of my patients in cardiac arrest from hyperkalemia were treated this way. All three of them got a pulse back. All three of them were treated with dialysis. All three recovered completely. All three were discharged from the hospital and were able to hug their family members again, share more laughs and create more memories.

As an ER doc, there is no feeling more incredible than the pure exhilaration of snatching a patient from the jaws of death and saving his or her life. I've always thought that must be what it feels like to win a Super Bowl. All the studying, the hard work, countless nights without sleep in the hospital and the singular devotion to learning your craft and honing your skills provide the framework that enables you to immediately diagnose and effectively treat a condition that would otherwise have killed your patient.

The weight of that responsibility is crushing at times, but when you pull it off, there is no better feeling.

CHAPTER SIX

House Doc

After completing an internship, a physician sits for Step III of boards, the final test to obtain a medical license. You still need to finish residency and pass your specialty boards, but once you have a medical license, your horizons become broader with regard to medical practice. In my residency, obtaining your license to practice medicine independently meant two important things: you could start to fly on the Life Flight helicopter, and you could moonlight. One moonlighting opportunity in our hospital was working as the "House Doc," which meant taking call to cover the patients who had been admitted by private attendings and were not covered by the other resident services.

It was during a House Doc call shift that I first applied my training to improvise in the treatment of a critically ill patient.

I was called to the bedside of a 72-year-old woman with congestive heart failure. She was becoming increasingly short of breath, and you could hear rales, or crackles, most of the way up her chest. She could not lay back due to feeling that she was suffocating when she did so, a medical symptom called orthopnea. Her oxygen saturation level was still acceptable, but unless she improved quickly, she would undoubtedly require intubation and mechanical ventilation.

As an ER resident, every chance to intubate a patient was welcome purely from a skill development perspective, but I wanted to avoid intubating this patient, in part because it was always challenging to intubate patients with severe pulmonary edema (too much fluid in their lungs). They strongly resisted being laid back. We often addressed this by performing nasal intubation with the patient sitting up. Later in my residency, the technique of RSI (rapid sequence intubation), consisting of giving medications to induce a state of deep sedation then paralyzing the patient, was shown to improve the odds of successfully intubating a patient on the first attempt. At the time, however, it was always a struggle to intubate these patients without having them decompensate, sometimes dangerously.

This patient needed intravenous medications including nitroglycerin, furosemide and morphine. Only one problem: the patient didn't have any IV access, and the nurses couldn't find a vein. I needed to place a central line, a large-bore IV that goes directly into one of the big veins in your neck, chest or groin. I had never placed a central line in a patient who was sitting up, though, and there was no way I could wrestle her flat onto her back.

I recalled studying a technique that just might work if I could do it with the patient sitting up. I referred to my pocket guidebook that described how to do procedures and quickly reviewed how to place a subclavian central line using a supraclavicular approach. In other words, I stood at the patient's side with a huge needle pointed toward her chest while coming in from above her collar bone. I'd never done it before. I'd never seen it done. I didn't have time to ask anyone if they thought it was a good idea.

As I slid the needle under her clavicle, I saw the flash of blood that told me I was in a blood vessel, which was a good start. I drew back the plunger to confirm more blood return, then removed the syringe, slid the guide wire into her vein without meeting resistance, removed the metal needle and slid the soft catheter over the guide wire in a series of steps known as a modified Seldinger technique.

The entire procedure went smoothly, and within minutes the patient had a triple lumen central venous catheter through which I gave her diuretics, nitro and morphine aggressively. She responded beautifully and was feeling better within an hour of my having been called to her bedside, avoiding intubation.

For the first time, I was able to improvise because I understood all the pieces and how they needed to come together in order to act decisively; everything went just as I envisioned it. It was a win-win: for the patient, and for me.

CHAPTER SEVEN

Learning My Way

The learning curve of a medical education is steep and involves several transitions that pose new, exciting, and sometimes terrifying challenges.

The first huge transition in medical school occurs when moving from the second to third years. Reading about diseases is replaced with talking to patients and trying to figure out which ones they have. Theories about how to treat disease are translated on paper as you write orders for tests and therapies for patients.

The second transition, from medical school to residency, is even more difficult, as you begin to make decisions on your own and become more directly responsible for patient care. You still have plenty of backup as you complete various rotations relevant to your specialty, but you're flying solo for the first time.

A typical first year of an emergency medicine residency includes rotations in pediatrics, internal medicine, cardiology, anesthesiology, trauma surgery, OB/GYN and a rotation or two in the ER. The second year adds neurology, neurosurgery, more trauma, ICU rotations and more time in the ER. The third year includes rotations such as EMS, more ICU time, an elective, and several months in the ER.

Each year better prepares you to function on your own in the ER. An amusing but understandable phenomenon occurs at some point in your last year of residency: the confidence you have built to that point becomes shaky as you start to realize you will be on your own soon. Do you know everything you need to know? This is particularly intimidating in emergency medicine because anything can come through the doors at any time, and there is no possible way to prepare for every contingency.

In my experience, though, the most challenging transition as an ER doctor was my first year or two after residency. After years of having backup and support at nearly every turn, all responsibility as an attending emergency physician now fell on me on Day 1.

I learned some of the most important lessons of my career during the first couple of years after completing my residency in emergency medicine.

Chief complaint: "Flank pain"

A 52-year-old man presented with sudden onset of right flank pain. He looked like he had a kidney stone. He acted like he had a kidney stone. He had blood in his urine like a kidney stone. He was concerned, though, because three months prior his twin brother had been diagnosed with renal cell carcinoma: kidney cancer.

Relying on my mere months of experience, I told him I didn't think he had to worry about having kidney cancer for two reasons. One, his presentation was classic for a kidney stone. Everything fit. Sudden onset of severe flank pain, a benign abdominal exam and hematuria (blood in the urine). Kidney stone. Book it.

Two, the odds of twin brothers being diagnosed with renal cell carcinoma a few months apart in their fifties was extraordinarily unlikely.

Just a note about kidney stones: they suck! From an emergency medicine standpoint, a kidney stone is not the most difficult thing to diagnose. At times you can look at a patient checking in at the front desk on the security camera and see the patient doing the "kidney stone dance" and diagnose it from there. The reputation of how painful kidney stones are is well-deserved. I've had women who have given natural childbirth and had a kidney stone tell me that the kidney stone was worse! "At least with contractions you get a minute or two of relief in between. The pain from a kidney stone is constant," some say. Others have said childbirth without any pain medications is definitely worse. The fact that this is even a conversation should convince you they really do suck.

I ordered the usual for a kidney stone patient: a CT scan, something for nausea, and most importantly, pain medication.

His CT showed renal cell carcinoma.

Oh. My. God.

Lesson learned: Don't make unnecessary predictions.

Why had I said *anything*? It didn't need to be said. I had already ordered the test that would provide the diagnosis. I should have told him we'd have some answers soon. Why had I felt the need to provide commentary, or demonstrate my prowess at making predictions like I was Nostradamus? I felt like an idiot.

This was an unforced error. I had fulfilled my primary objectives: I relieved his pain and I reached an accurate diagnosis. I didn't miss something or get anything "wrong." While it would have been devastating to inform him and his wife that he had cancer anyway, my needless and, in the end, false reassurance only made it worse.

I stopped trying to predict the future long ago.

Interestingly, in my first two years out of residency I had three patients who presented precisely like a kidney stone who had renal cell carcinoma. I was ultra-paranoid about any patient with flank pain for years. It turned out to be an extraordinarily unlikely cluster of patients with a relatively rare diagnosis, thankfully.

Chief complaint: "Trouble walking"

A 24-year-old male presents to the ER with a somewhat unusual complaint. He noticed he seemed to be having trouble walking, but he wasn't exactly sure why. He didn't feel weak per se, nor did he feel sick at all. He'd been completely fine except for a cold he had gotten over about a week ago. He hadn't had any problems controlling his bowel or bladder, hadn't noticed any problems with his strength in his hands, nor had any numbness or tingling in his arms or legs.

His exam was unremarkable except for two subtle but significant findings. He had normal reflexes at the knees, but none at the ankles. He seemed to have normal strength when I tested him while he was sitting, and also when he got up to walk. When I asked him to walk on his toes, however, he couldn't do it. It's not normal for a healthy 24-year-old not to be able to walk on his toes.

There were no other tests I needed to perform, nothing else that could help me immediately determine what was wrong with him. This was a clinical diagnosis, the type that is made only by suspecting the problem and by having enough medical knowledge of the disease process to feel comfortable in diagnosing it.

I was fairly confident that my patient had Guillain-Barré syndrome, a rare neurologic disorder that can follow a viral illness. The cause is unknown, and the treatments are rudimentary at best. Guillain-Barré causes ascending paralysis; weakness starts in the feet and can spread all the way up the body to the point that the patient is paralyzed, including the muscles that allow you to breathe.

Knowing this, I made a call to the patient's internist.

"Hi Doctor Johnson, this is Reggie Duling from the ER. Say, I have a patient of yours named Paul Ramirez: he's a 24-year-old otherwise healthy man who presents today with what I am concerned is Guillain-Barré syndrome."

I saw this patient about six weeks after graduating from residency. I am sure Dr. Johnson was aware of this, and on the other end of the phone he probably rolled his eyes before responding.

"Really? Well, tell him to come to my office later this week."

I wondered if he had heard me correctly. The patient clearly needed to be hospitalized.

"Well, um, he needs to be hospitalized in case he gets worse. Doesn't he?"

There it was: doubt creeping in. Not his; mine. Of course, Dr. Johnson doubted me! The neophyte doctor who finished residency six weeks ago and is scared shitless that he might miss something thinks he has a Guillain-Barré patient? Do you know how rare that is? How unlikely?

He responded again, "So what are you saying?"

"I'm saying I think he needs to be admitted and evaluated by a neurologist."

"Fine," Dr. Johnson said, obviously perturbed but not wanting to get into it with me. "Send him to my office right now and I'll take care of him."

It sounded like an odd approach, but I had just finished seven years of medical training during which when an attending physician tells you to do something, the discussion is over. I thought to myself, "That's fine. I'll send the patient over, then *you* will see what *I* see."

Two days later I decided to follow up on the patient, but I couldn't find him anywhere in the hospital. I called his home number to check up on him. I talked to his friend, George, who had been with him in the ER two days prior.

"How is Paul doing?"

"He's in the hospital."

"I looked for him in the hospital. I couldn't find him."

"He's at another hospital."

"What do you mean? How did he get to another hospital?"

"When we left the ER, we went to see Dr. Johnson like you told us. He took a look at Paul and told him he was fine and sent him home. The next day he woke up and couldn't breathe, so I had to call 911. He is on a ventilator."

I instantly felt sick to my stomach. I was dumbfounded, and instantly angry: at Dr. Johnson, but more at myself. Why hadn't I insisted that he be admitted to the hospital from the ER?

Lesson learned: Trust your own judgement.

This was a facet of being an ER doc it took me some time to learn. As a resident you operate in a mode of deference. If an attending tells you to do something, you do it. You might ask why you're doing something, but you never really questioned whether it was the right thing to do.

The day you graduate from residency and are on your own, you are expected to be the one who knows what's right. In Paul's case, I did most of the things that could have been expected of a physician. I listened to his history. I performed a thorough physical examination that revealed subtle but significant findings. Truth be told, it was actually a pretty astute pick-up on my part. I correctly identified a zebra, an uncommon but potentially dangerous condition.

My error was substituting another physician's judgment for my own merely because he'd been practicing medicine longer than me. I was the one who talked to the patient, examined the patient, given thought to his condition and developed a differential diagnosis. What was Dr. Johnson basing his opposition to my diagnosis on? To immediately dismiss my concerns actually required an unhealthy level of arrogance on Dr. Johnson's part. This is not an uncommon phenomenon in emergency medicine. A doctor you just woke up at 3 a.m. to admit a patient thinks they are able to determine in 30 seconds that what you're telling them must be wrong without having looked at the chart or the patient.

Learning not to defer to what other physicians tell you is a critical part of practicing medicine. Learning to trust your own instincts and knowledge is imperative. The balance is delicate, though, because you also have to learn to question yourself and allow for the possibility that *you* could be wrong. The balance between humility and confidence as a doctor is delicate, as both are indispensable.

Chief complaint: Rash

A 76-year-old man presents with a rash on his face. I'll spare you the suspense. He had zoster, or shingles. It was classic. The rash covered his left upper cheek and was around his eye, as well as the left side of his nose and the left side of his forehead. He didn't have Hutchinson's sign, a shingles lesion on the tip of the nose, which can indicate ocular involvement, as shingles can infect your cornea. The patient didn't have eye pain, which he almost certainly would have had with zoster keratitis, but I believe in being thorough. If there is one thing I've tried hard never to do in my medical career, it is to miss something out of laziness. It's easier and smarter to just check on whatever it is you're thinking about it, then you don't have to worry about it again. As such, I stained his left eye with fluorescein and examined his cornea under the slit lamp, a piece of equipment used to obtain a magnified view of the eye. I looked for dendritic lesions that would indicate corneal involvement of his shingles. He didn't have any. I was satisfied.

His wife had made an offhand comment that he'd seemed a bit confused earlier. I didn't quite dismiss it. I asked him about it. I hadn't detected any problem while talking to him. He carried on a conversation normally and seemed sharp when answering my questions. His wife also admitted that he didn't seem confused at that moment. He said he was fine and had no idea why she was worried.

Three days later he was found to have zoster encephalitis, a rare but dangerous complication created by the virus causing inflammation of the brain.

Lesson learned: Always listen for subtle clues.

I couldn't blame this on deferring to a consultant. I am not sure I would have been convinced to do a lumbar puncture (spinal tap) at the time, but I probably would have given him more careful discharge instructions, telling him to return immediately if either the patient or his wife were concerned about anything.

Chief complaint: My potassium is high

A 64-year-old woman presents after she was called by her primary care physician and told to come to the ER right away. She had labs drawn at her doctor's office yesterday and it was just discovered that her potassium level was "dangerously high" at 6.7.

The patient was completely freaked out, convinced she could die. Her daughter drove her to the ER and the daughter is panicked as well.

You may recall the significance of hyperkalemia, a high potassium level. As I interviewed her, though, I learned that she had no history of kidney problems, took no potassium-sparing diuretics, ACE inhibitors, ARBs, was not diabetic, and was not on a potassium supplement; she had no reason to have a dangerously high potassium level. Accordingly, I ordered the only test I needed: a repeat potassium level.

Potassium is stored in our cells. Sometimes drawing blood causes hemolysis, when red blood cells break open, releasing their potassium, which is now measured at a higher level in serum than it actually is. The condition is called pseudohyperkalemia, or "false" hyperkalemia.

The recheck of her potassium was 4.3, completely normal.

Lesson learned: If something doesn't sound right, question it.

Another example I've seen a few times is when all the blood cell lines are low. Your white blood cell count is low (leukopenia), your red blood cell count is low (anemia), and your platelet count is low (thrombo-cytopenia). This can occur as part of a very serious medical condition in which your bone marrow isn't producing blood cells normally. However, it also may be that your blood was drawn off an IV line through which fluid was running, so that a tiny bit of the IV fluid was drawn up with the blood, diluting everything you test for, making all the values lower than normal.

My most memorable illustration of the importance of questioning results before acting on them occurred after

I saw a female patient with symptoms of a urinary tract infection. I sent a urine sample to the lab to confirm my suspicion. As expected, her urine looked infected. Easy enough. Except the lab report also commented that sperm were present. This isn't unheard of in the ER. Things that bring people to the ER happen at all times of the day or night under all sorts of circumstances, one of them being having recently had sex.

I called the lab and spoke with the lab tech.

"I want to double check this result. You commented that sperm were present."

"Yes?" he asked more than affirmed, as he usually didn't get a call from the ER for this kind of result.

"Can you double check that? I need to be absolutely certain that is what you are seeing."

"We see it all the time. What's the big deal?" he asked innocently.

"This patient is five years old."

A 25-year-old woman with a UTI and sperm in her urine? I wouldn't give it another thought. A 5-year-old girl? That opens a gigantic can of worms. Jumping to conclusions based on an erroneous result would be disastrous. Even worse, missing or ignoring a legitimate result such as this would be abhorrent.

After taking a second look, he apologized and said there was no way they were sperm.

Can you imagine if I had taken that result to be fact and acted on it? I'm pretty sure kicking the door in and storming into the patient's room and yelling at the father, "I just called CPS and the cops, you piece of shit!" would not have gone over well when all the facts were known.

Abdominal Pain of Undetermined Etiology

Many patients come to the ER with abdominal pain because they want to know one thing: do they have appendicitis?

Answer: it can be really hard to tell, especially in the first few to several hours of symptoms. Initial symptoms can include vague pain around the belly button, which is not the classic location for abdominal pain in appendicitis.

Symptoms may include nausea, vomiting, fever, chills and loss of appetite. Sound like any illness you've ever had? Of course it does! It sounds like almost *every* illness.

We know full well that if you present with abdominal pain of three hours' duration, there's a chance that you have early appendicitis, but there's no good way to figure it out this early in the disease process. Your blood work may be completely normal, and your CT might not show anything yet, so we give it time. We tell you to come back within 24 hours so we can take a second look at you, see if your labs have changed, reexamine your belly to determine if the location and nature of your pain are more convincing, and likely to obtain a CT, which is far more likely to yield a diagnosis.

Lesson learned: Prepare yourself and the patient for the fact that conditions change.

If you've ever been an ER patient, you've undoubtedly been told to come back if your symptoms get worse. We want to prepare you for the possibility that what you have could be more serious and require further attention, but it's just too early to know, so we tell you that if your symptoms get worse, you feel sicker, or you are concerned, you should come back so we can take a second look.

Chief complaint: Knee pain

An 82-year-old woman presents with knee pain. Both knees had bothered her for years but had become more painful recently. There was nothing remarkable about her physical exam—no signs of infection or something more sinister. I ordered x-rays, which showed severe arthritis, not surprising given her age and chronic knee pain. Straightforward case, which was always welcome.

Not wanting to prescribe narcotics to an 82-year-old, which would likely only cause confusion, difficulty performing her daily activities, and potentially severe constipation, I told her to use Tylenol or ibuprofen. They're both over-the-counter medications.

A week later, I learned that she was in the intensive care unit and was not expected to survive. She'd been admitted with an exacerbation of her chronic heart failure, pulmonary edema, and kidney failure.

Most likely, her heart failure had worsened, decreasing perfusion to her kidneys, resulting in acute kidney injury.

It was also possible, though, that she had taken too much ibuprofen, a nonsteroidal anti-inflammatory drug. NSAIDs can cause kidney failure if taken in too high of doses or for too long, and dysfunction of her kidneys could have precipitated fluid overload and decompensated heart failure.

Lesson learned: Nothing in medicine is risk-free.

Every day, doctors perform invasive procedures with potential for dangerous complications, and prescribe medications that could have deleterious side effects. You cram so many goddam facts in your head trying not to miss something, yet medicine and the human body are so complicated that the reality is that you could potentially cause harm even with an offhand comment to take some Tylenol or ibuprofen.

The Perfect Score

I once interviewed a gentleman who told me he had just passed his recertification exam in emergency medicine, which is required every ten years.

"I passed by one point. The perfect score," he bragged.

I laughed it off in the moment, understanding the bottom-line mentality of it, but over the next couple of days I kept thinking about it, and it bothered me more and more. Sure, it was a casual comment that was probably intended to be humorous, but what kind of attitude was that about medicine?

Lesson learned: Be a lifelong learner.

The most frightening part of being an ER doc is never knowing what's coming through those doors next. A 25-week premature breech delivery? That patient makes an experienced obstetrician nervous in a hospital with all kinds of backup available. To an ER doctor who hasn't delivered a baby since their OB/GYN rotation in residency, and has not once had to handle such an obstetric emergency? It raises the old sphincter tone, to say the least.

No matter how much you know, study, practice, rehearse or visualize, there are countless scenarios that will challenge or potentially exceed your abilities. The only way to combat the fear is to never stop learning, so that if you fail to respond to a challenge when your name is called, you can live with the fact that you did everything you could.

I strongly believe that we should never stop learning in life. We should constantly strive to become better people, better husbands, wives, fathers, mothers, sons, daughters, friends, colleagues, and yes, doctors or whatever else it is that we do. We'll never achieve perfection, but the pursuit of our best should be embraced and celebrated. We should recognize in each other the effort put forth, and when our best might not be good enough, as will happen to all of us many times during our journey, we should extend a little empathy.

A Lesson Learned on Television

The television show *ER* premiered during my fourth year of medical school in the fall of 1994. The show was a smash hit with audiences across the country from the start, perhaps with none more than the group of medical students and doctors who had chosen to become emergency physicians.

I was in the process of applying to emergency medicine residencies at the time. I followed the show as closely as I could, vicariously experiencing what my life would soon resemble.

In March of 1995, I eagerly stood with my classmates on Match Day, waiting for my name to be called and the envelope handed to me that contained the name of the emergency medicine residency program I would be joining in July.

That same month, an episode of ER titled "Love's Labor Lost" aired. In it, Dr. Mark Greene, the heart and soul of the series for many years, treated a pregnant patient for what initially seemed like a minor ailment.

The patient decompensated over time, however, and Dr. Greene couldn't get anyone to help him. Spoiler Alert! As a last resort, Dr. Greene performed an emergent C-section. The baby survived, but the mother suddenly decompensated and died.

The episode was devastating to everyone who watched it, I'm sure, but as someone who was about to start training to become like Dr. Greene, this episode of a television show intended to entertain the masses somehow left an indelible mark on my psyche.

Years later, as the actor Anthony Edwards' run on the show neared its end, Dr. Greene was diagnosed with a brain tumor. He died during an episode aired in May of 2002. By that time, I'd been through residency and had been a practicing ER doc for four years.

It felt like a colleague had died. The character of Mark Greene epitomized what any ER doctor should hope to be: deeply caring, clinically astute, imperfectly human.

Lesson learned: I've been fortunate enough to know a lot of Mark Greenes.

CHAPTER EIGHT

A Rite of Passage

Medicine, like most vocations that require constant interaction with the public, introduces you to some real characters. In residency, one of the most compelling was Dr. Gordon Canfield.

Gordon only worked nights at the busiest ER in the city. Legend held that he'd been a combat medic in Vietnam and liked it so much it drove him to become an ER doctor. He was a cantankerous guy who seemed older than he was, in part because he had a deep, leathery tan of his face and neck from tending to his orchards all day before coming in to work the night shift. I have no idea when Gordon slept.

Dr. Canfield was a legend among the residents. First, he used to teach a lesson on ballistics and gunshot wounds by taking the residents to his private property and having them shoot an assortment of weaponry. Second, he got away with things for which he'd be fired instantly by today's standards. Third, he didn't particularly like residents; at least residents who were slow, or who created more work for him. Our residency was based in two busy community ERs: the mother ship and Gordon's. No one worked with Gordon until you were deemed ready as a second-year resident; no interns were allowed to work with Gordon.

It was a rite of passage when you were signed off to work night shifts with Dr. Canfield. It was a confidence booster when you got the feeling that he approved of you, which was hard to get a read on, mostly because if your shift went well, you might never see him.

Whenever he wasn't needed to keep the ER running, Dr. Canfield spent his time doing two things: chain-smoking and reloading ammunition shells—at the same time. I still have no idea how that was even remotely a good idea, smoking while working with gunpowder. He had a reloader on his desk. It seemed he spent a lot of time doing it, but maybe that's because you rarely dared to go back to Gordon's office. As one of my attendings put it, "Every time I leave Gordon's office, I think I should get a chest x-ray."

Dr. Canfield also spoke in a muffled, gruff voice that was hard to hear and understand. During a typical night shift, patient arrivals would finally subside to a number you could handle alone, and off he'd go to supply the world with cigarette butts and ammo.

Invariably, things would pick up, and once again you'd be overwhelmed with patients. As this was in the days before large computer monitors were mounted on the wall as patient trackers, we had a large number of paper facesheets on clipboards hanging on the wall. As you signed up for the next patient, you put your initials on the facesheet to indicate that patient was already being seen. As you fell further behind, more blank facesheets accumulated on the wall. You'd exit a patient's room and head to the board where Gordon was standing. "They're coming in under the wire," he'd mutter before putting his initials on several facesheets. He'd bail you out, then silently vanish back to his den.

Gordon's personality was, shall we say, more confrontational at times. I once tried to admit a patient to urology and was getting pushback from the urology resident. Gordon came over and spoke briefly to the resident but was similarly rebuked. He said, "Are you listening to me?" then he repeatedly slammed the phone down on the desk hard before putting the receiver back to his ear. "Get down here right now and see the patient." The patient was admitted.

A young male patient who clearly knew how the system worked made the mistake of using a tone that implied Gordon was like a waiter taking his order. "Go get the social worker. I need a voucher to fill my prescription." Gordon turned around, walked out to the nurses' station, located a phone book, and within a minute or so he marched back into the patient's room. He had ripped a sheet out of the Yellow Pages which he now jammed into the patient's pocket. "Here you go," Gordon grunted. "That's a list of pawn shops. You can go sell your gold chain and pay for your own prescription."

My favorite encounter was brief and direct. A 19-year-old came in claiming to be paralyzed from the waist down after he'd been using a Ouija board. The patient had brought the Ouija board with him as though it were evidence of his curse. Upon hearing this, Dr. Canfield briskly entered the room and angrily told the patient, "We've got a lot of sick patients here and we need this bed. If you don't get up and walk out of here, I'm going to shove that Ouija board up your ass! Now get out!" The patient miraculously walked out.

Dr. Gordon Canfield was colorful to say the least. Sadly, chain-smoking, playing with guns, excessive sun exposure, burning the candle at both ends, not sleeping and working nights caught up with him, and Dr. Canfield died in his 50's.

To paraphrase Walt Whitman, he was a memorable character in this powerful play who contributed a verse.

CHAPTER NINE

Medicine in the Wild Blue Yonder

Hands down, the most exciting part of finishing internship and obtaining a medical license was the opportunity to serve as a physician on the Life Flight helicopter. I became a medic in the Army almost ten years after the last American troops left Vietnam, so there were plenty of senior NCOs and officers around who had served there. While Vietnam vets were treated horribly by civilians, among us troops they were heroes and legends. For those of us in the medical field, perhaps none more than MedEvac pilots, crew and medics.

Occasionally, during field exercises, I was able to hitch a ride or two on an old Huey, a Bell UH-1 Iroquois helicopter. They had a very distinctive sound and became synonymous with the Vietnam War. During my time on Active Duty, Hueys were being phased out in favor of the UH-60 Black Hawk, but it was easy to romanticize how badass the Huey was and what it must have been like to serve as part of a flight crew in Vietnam. I suppose it's easy to romanticize something you've never experienced, especially when no one is shooting at you.

Aeromedical transports come in two flavors: interhospital transfers and scene flights. Most MedEvac flights are interhospital transfers, taking a sick or injured patient from one hospital to another that can provide a higher level of care. Sometimes these patients are

66

relatively stable, needing only someone to monitor them closely until they arrive at the destination medical facility. Other times the patient barely made it to the outside hospital and needed to get out of there as quickly as possible to give them any chance at survival.

I loved everything about flying, from the smell of jet fuel to the sound of the turbine engines to the silhouette of our Dauphin helicopter against the sky. I loved putting on my flight suit and my name tag embroidered with wings. All us residents loved flight shifts. Knee-deep in patients in the ER, once the flight beeper sounded, I handed my patients off to the attending physicians and headed to the helipad, excited about what adventure might await.

One such adventure yielded my first and only opportunity to "crack a chest." A 37-year-old man had been in a collision, car vs train. As our flight crew entered the ER, I heard the attending ER doc say, "We've lost a pulse. Let's crack his chest."

"Holy cow!" I thought to myself. I'd wanted to see one of these done in real time since I first learned about them. I'd practiced the technique in pig labs and rehearsed it in my head many times. I was hoping to get a closer look when the attending physician looked right at me and said, "You ever done one of these?"

I responded truthfully, "No."

"Well, come on. You're about to."

Gulp.

A resuscitative thoracotomy, by its technical term, consists of making a quick incision from the sternum down the left side of the chest until your hand hits the bed with purpose, ensuring you cut deep enough to enter the chest cavity. Or, as it was taught to me, "cut the patient like you mean it." A rib spreader is then used to pry two ribs apart so that the heart and lung are exposed. The pericardium, the sac that surrounds the heart, is opened with scissors to relieve tamponade, pressure caused by bleeding within the pericardium, and to expose the heart itself so that any holes caused by gunshot or stab wounds can be plugged. From there, the aorta is located running behind the heart in front of the spine, and the aorta is "cross-clamped." This is done to keep all blood flow going north to the head and neck in an attempt to maintain perfusion of the brain.

A resuscitative thoracotomy is attempted as a last resort. It rarely works, particularly on blunt trauma patients. If you are stabbed in the heart and lose vital signs, cracking your chest might allow the doctor to relieve the pressure around your heart by releasing a pericardial tamponade, then stop the bleeding by inserting a foley catheter, which is normally used to drain your bladder, through the hole in your heart, then blowing up the balloon at the end of the foley and pulling it tightly against the inside wall of your heart. Basically, relieve the pressure, plug the hole, then hope you can restart the heart.

For blunt trauma, though, the cause of death is less likely to be something you can fix by cracking a chest, but when a young life is on the line, you try everything possible.

"Nice work!" the attending physician said encouragingly as I finished cross-clamping the aorta.

We continued the attempt at resuscitation, but in the end the patient's trauma was too great to overcome, and the attending ER doc pronounced him dead.

The attending physician was a graduate of my residency program and had loved flying as much as I did. I found it quite reassuring to have an ally in our fight against death. He was also looking out for me, offering guidance and support as we performed this incredible intervention together. The patient had died, but on the flight home I felt satisfied knowing I had done everything I possibly could, employing my skill and knowledge to the best of my ability.

Sometimes, though, doing your best feels empty and meaningless, and all you can think about is the tragedy and loss. Such was the case after a flight in the middle of a cold night in January. When the Life Flight beeper chirped, always a welcome sound, I gleefully strode to the chopper and embarked.

Upon landing, we were escorted into the ER in a small town with an ER that only appeared to have one patient. We were directed to the bedside where a young doctor and the ER staff were performing CPR. I feared we'd arrived too late and was aghast when I looked to see that the patient was a baby.

In a nightmarish scenario that has haunted my dreams, a new mother had been nursing her baby in a recliner. At some point, the exhausted mom fell asleep and awoke to find that her baby had slid off her chest headfirst into a wastebasket next to her recliner. As the baby was head-down, too weak to control its head and neck or even to cry out, the child suffocated.

The physician on duty in the small community hospital was an internal medicine resident who was in his second year of training, just as I was. Many residents liked to moonlight in addition to their residency training, myself included. Moonlighting allowed you to make some extra money and, more importantly, to gain valuable real-world experience making medical decisions on your own. You never bargained for something like this, though.

I couldn't imagine how terrifying that must have been for him. Internal medicine doctors train to care for adult patients only. They don't do pediatric rotations beyond their medical school training. Despite his lack of training in peds, however, he had performed admirably. He intubated the infant and placed an intraosseous line, a hollow needle drilled into the tibia bone on the lower leg to provide access to deliver medications. He had run through the appropriate PALS (Pediatric Advanced Life Support) algorithms but had no response.

After I arrived at the bedside, we ran through a couple more rounds of PALS together, though I had little to offer except reassurance that he had done everything I could think of to do. I could tell it rattled him. How could it not? The flight crew stuck around as he told the mother. There are few emotional experiences in life as devastating as a mother's grief. The flight home was quiet as the flight crew contemplated what we'd just seen. I was not yet a father, but completely understood when the flight nurse said over the headset that she just wanted to get home to hug her kids.

Fortunately, most interhospital transfers were not nearly as traumatic.

The other type of MedEvac was the scene flight—the chopper was called to the scene of what was almost always a trauma case. For adrenaline junkies like ER doctors, scene flights were exhilarating.

Life Flight helicopters served as critical care transport vehicles. At times, inclement weather grounded the helicopter, and we had to travel by ground transport. I once rode two hours in our ambulance with a young woman who had stood too close to an industrial machine which literally tore her entire scalp off in one piece. We transported her through the ice and snow to the University of Michigan, where they reattached her scalp.

While flying was tremendous fun and one of the primary reasons I decided to return to my hometown for residency, as one prone to motion sickness under the wrong conditions, I did almost puke my guts out once.

Called to transfer a patient from a Detroit hospital, by the time we arrived in the Detroit airspace, a dense fog had settled on the area. Life Flight pilots were instrument-rated, but they still had to be able to see the hospital at some point, and on this day the pilot was unable to locate it. With nothing to focus on outside the aircraft but fog, what seemed like endless swerving, banking and circling made me question just how cool being a flight physician was after all.

"Jesus, are we in a dogfight?!" I wanted to yell at the pilot. Instead, I focused all my energy on my nausea and my attempt not to hurl all over the inside of the helicopter.

Months later, on a gorgeous spring day, I took in the breathtaking landscapes on our way to the scene of a boating accident. The pilot gently set the chopper down close to an idyllic lake in southern Michigan. We deboarded the aircraft and walked to the back of a waiting ambulance where the patient, a 12-year-old boy, was lying on a gurney.

The doors of the ambulance were open to face the lake, as well as a sizable crowd of onlookers. The boy had been tubing behind his family's boat when the tow rope snapped. As the boy spun around on the inner tube, the rope recoiled sharply, impaling a thick, metal S-hook through his skull. It was attached to a small buoy which could not be detached with any tools available at the lakeside, so the rope attached to the buoy had been cut.

I climbed into the back of the ambulance and moved to the patient's head where I could fully visualize the pigtail of rope connected to the buoy and in turn the S-hook, half of which was embedded in the boy's skull.

He was initially awake, alert, and answered a couple of questions appropriately, but he soon became increasingly confused. Suddenly, he became more agitated, and began screaming profanities, a clear sign that his mental status was rapidly deteriorating due to increased intracranial pressure. He began thrashing about violently as he became combative and had to be held down. This was the worst thing possible for his head injury. I needed to keep him still and quiet, and the only way to do that was to sedate, paralyze and intubate him.

Rapid sequence intubation had recently become the preferred technique for airway management. I'd performed RSI in the ER under the watchful eye of my attending physician, but this was my first opportunity to utilize the technique on my own. The Life Flight nurse drew up the medications into syringes and helped me prepare the equipment we would need.

The flight nurse pushed the drugs as I ordered them.

"Lidocaine 50 mg IV push."

"Given."

"Fentanyl 35 micrograms IV."

"Given."

"Vecuronium 0.4 mg IV."

"Given."

"Etomidate 20 mg IV push."

"Given."

"Succinylcholine 70 mg IV."

"Given."

As the medications were given in quick succession, the boy stopped talking, and as the succinylcholine, a paralytic agent, took effect, his body relaxed completely. Now it was all on me. Succinylcholine worked for 4–6 minutes before wearing off, just enough time to get the tube in and start delivering oxygen before brain cells started to die.

I'd done over a hundred intubations by this point in my residency, though not many had been done on kids. Ignoring this fact, I visualized his vocal cords and slid the endotracheal tube between them to the proper depth, which was determined by the formula "4 + age/4," which for this 12-year-old boy meant using a size 7 ET tube. I inflated the cuff and began to bag him. I confirmed tube placement, secured the tube, and urged the flight nurse, "Let's get him loaded up and out of here."

We flew him back to our level I Trauma Center where he underwent surgery to remove the tow hook.

My experiences on Life Flight were a vital part of learning to apply all the medical knowledge and skills I'd acquired to that point to save lives. There was nothing like it.

The helicopter was also one of my favorite places to reflect. On the flight home after delivering a patient, there usually wasn't a lot of chatter. The muffled whoop-whoop-whoop of the rotor blades on our Dauphin provided calming white noise. One morning right at dawn we were headed north on our way back from a long flight to Columbus. At one perfect moment, you could look out the west side of the aircraft and see the dark, night sky, while out the east window the sun beamed through a clear blue sky indicating that the day had begun. The sight was mesmerizing. That day epitomized much of what the ER is all about: brief periods of intense focus and performance followed by down time you have to take advantage of by appreciating the beauty in life.

CHAPTER TEN

Jerry Springer Moments

Chief complaint: "I need to be checked for STDs."

A 24-year-old male presents to the emergency department stating, "I need to be checked for STDs." This is not an uncommon complaint in the ER, but I found it a bit unusual to find out that the woman sitting next to him was his wife. After asking a couple of questions, it was clear that his wife had dragged him in after he had cheated on her. She was the next to speak.

"He needs to be checked for gonorrhea, chlamydia, and herpes," his wife pronounced very matter-of-factly.

I was curious why she was concerned about those in particular. Were those STDs she had heard of? She wasn't concerned about syphilis or HIV?

I asked, "Why are you concerned about those diseases in particular?"

"Because that's what he was exposed to!" she snapped back at me, as if I was supposed to have known that already.

As this conversation was occurring, the nurse was in the room as well, and we occasionally exchanged glances as this ever-more-interesting story unfolded.

"Well, how would you know what he was exposed to?" I inquired.

One mark of a professional is that no matter how bizarre or unexpected something is, act as if the response is completely expected and normal. I again glanced at the nurse as we both anticipated her answer.

"Because he slept with my sister, and that's what she has."

Chief complaint: Abdominal pain

A fourteen-year-old girl complained of right upper quadrant abdominal pain. As part of obtaining a complete history I asked other fairly routine questions.

"Any fever?" I asked.

"No."

"Vomiting or diarrhea?"

"Nope."

"Does it hurt or burn when you urinate?"

"Nuh uh."

"Are you urinating more often than you normally do, or does it feel like you have to go to the bathroom all the time?"

"No."

"Have you had any sort of vaginal discharge?"

Now, when I ask that question of most fourteen-year-olds, I usually get an odd look as if they have no idea what I am talking about, which is understandable. She was able to tell me right off the bat, though.

"A little."

"What color is it?" I asked.

"I'm not sure."

I could have left it at that, but in trying to be thorough, I figured I'd make another run at it just to be sure. This is a learned skill in medicine; becoming an investigator. At times I feel as though I am interrogating then cross-examining patients to make sure we are on the same page. It is fairly common to get inaccurate responses from the first line of questioning. For example, if I ask a patient, "Are you a smoker?" and they tell me, "No," I follow it up with, "Have you ever smoked?" Why? Because people frequently say something like, "I quit last week," or "I quit after my heart attack last month." I am trying to ascertain their risk for smoking-related illnesses, but in their minds if they smoked three packs a day for thirty years but quit three days ago, they "don't smoke."

The same thing happens when asking about past medical problems.

"Do you have high blood pressure? Diabetes? High cholesterol?"

"No. No. No."

"Are you on medications?"

"Yes, I take atenolol (for blood pressure), Glucophage (for diabetes), and Lipitor (for cholesterol)."

If they're taking medication for the problem, many people figure it's no longer a problem.

Anyway, I couldn't just leave it alone, so I asked a question in an attempt to ensure that her vaginal discharge was not a sign of a pelvic infection. I hadn't even gotten to the touchy subject of whether or not she was sexually active.

I asked, "Is it clear? White? Yellow or green?"

She thought for a moment, then decided, "It's white."

That was good enough for me, but at this point her mother figured she'd help out by assisting me in clarifying this fact for the record. She did so by asking the following question, though it wasn't the actual question that bothered me so much as the tone, which was one that indicated she had every expectation that her fourteen-year-old daughter would know exactly what she was talking about.

"Is it cum-white?"

Chief complaint: Bumps down there

A twelve-year-old girl was brought in by her mother for "bumps down there." They had popped up a few days prior and were rather painful. She hadn't been particularly ill since the bumps appeared, but I was mildly surprised to learn that her mother was afraid she may have an STD. Mind you, I'd seen it all before: young girls getting pregnant soon after their first periods, child molestation at a young age, even STD's at this age.

Upon examining the patient, it was apparent that these "bumps" were in fact her first episode of genital herpes.

Her mother then asked, "How long does it take after you get herpes for the rash to appear?"

As I searched my memory banks for the incubation period of herpes, I asked her a question of my own.

"Why do you ask?"

"Well, I want to know which guy she got it from."

Wow! That said a lot: a twelve-year-old who wasn't sure which sexual partner she got it from, and her mom seemed just fine with it.

Her mother went on to explain that she had been with a twenty-year-old guy on Valentine's Day (how romantic), which had been about two months prior, and an older teen just about two weeks ago. After recalling that the incubation period for herpes was generally up to two weeks, with one week being the average, I told the patient's mom that it was more likely to be her more recent partner. The patient thought perhaps it had been the older guy, since her more recent partner had sex with her best friend on the same night he'd had sex with her, and as far as she knew her best friend was fine.

As far as I was concerned, it still sounded like a crime and a CPS referral. Hey, I'm the first to admit that being a parent isn't easy, but *daaaaaaaaamn*.

Nurse Consultant Call

A man called our nurse consulting line one night to ask if we could tell him how far mosquitoes fly. The first question that came to mind was, "Why would you want to know this?" It turned out he was planning a trip to Hawaii and wanted to know if mosquitoes could fly there from the West Coast, because he had seen on the news that mosquitoes carry West Nile virus, and he wanted to know if he needed to be concerned about infected mosquitoes making it to Hawaii from the mainland.

Chief complaint: "My vagina is broken."

A 45-year-old female presented to the ER stating, "The sticks that give my vagina its shape are all broken."

Having no idea what the hell she was talking about, I thought to myself, "This should be good."

She continued, "You know how normally there are two sticks on each side? Mine are all broken. I can push all four of them over to either side. They are also a lot lower than they were before."

I felt like I had completely missed the boat. Wanting to clarify things, I asked her to explain once again what the problem was.

"My vagina is broken!" she exclaimed. "I shouldn't be able to move it around like that."

I looked at her boyfriend, you know, man to man, trying to communicate with my eyes.

"Come on, buddy, how about a little help? You know that sounds batshit crazy, right?" my eyes pleaded.

The message was not received. Instead, he looked right at me and said, "Yeah, Doc. I've been with other women her age, and I'm not trying to be gross or nothin', but she has a very youthful vagina."

That's how he put it. She had a "very youthful vagina." What that meant exactly I had no idea, and I was sure I didn't want to know.

When I told them that I had no clue what they were talking about, they looked at me like *I* was stupid. Ultimately, her exam was normal, I tried to offer them both reassurance that I didn't see any problem, and she was on her way.

Chief complaint: "My feet are still bruised."

A 52-year-old male presented complaining that his feet were still bruised a month after he had sprained his ankles. He had no pain but was concerned about the black discoloration that remained around his ankles and extended all the way down to his toes.

As I examined his feet, I observed that both feet were affected similarly, which was unlikely for an injury. I also noticed that his feet felt rough, indicating that the black discoloration was on top of the skin rather than under the skin as bruising would be.

I went to the sink where I wetted a few 4x4 gauze pads, then began to rub them back and forth across the top of his left foot. While this seemed to have no effect at first, as I continued to apply a bit more pressure, after a couple of dozen strokes, I noticed that the black discoloration began to resolve, and with more vigorous scrubbing it disappeared completely.

The mystery was solved. The cause of the persistent black discoloration on both of the man's feet was…dirt.

Having demonstrated the cure for his affliction, I sent him home to complete the treatment in his bathtub.

CHAPTER ELEVEN

Can We Please Stop Referring to the Hippocratic Oath?

This is a lightly edited version of my article originally published in the
ACEP Medical Humanities Section Newsletter in July 2011

At the next committee meeting of The Powerful Who Decide Everything, I'd like to make a motion: Can we please stop referring to the Hippocratic Oath as the reason we do *anything* in medicine?

I'm as much of a traditionalist as the next doc, but I'm tired of hearing everyone from the press to the lay public to politicians to even other doctors telling me what I should and should not be doing because of the Hippocratic Oath.

First, I've never taken the Oath or any altered form of it, so stop telling me "You have to do this... or you can't do that... because you took the Hippocratic Oath." No, I didn't.

Second, most documents that are two millennia old are irrelevant and useless in the present day, like the Bible. Medicine was primitive, to put it kindly, one hundred years ago, back when the Joint Commission was telling field hospitals, "Keep your clean saws here and put your dirty saws over there. And don't forget to label your leeches."

Third, has anyone ever actually read the Hippocratic Oath our profession espouses to uphold? Here it is in italics, with my comments on each section.

I swear by Apollo the Physician and Asclepius and Hygeia and Panaceia and all the gods and goddesses, making them my witnesses, that I will fulfill according to my ability and judgment this oath and this covenant.

I don't swear anything by Apollo. I don't even use his name in vain, which is more than I can say for most gods.

To hold him who has taught me this art as equal to my parent and to live my life in partnership with him, and if he is in need of money to give him a share of mine, and to regard his offspring as equal to my brothers in male lineage and to teach them this art—if they desire to learn it—without fee and covenant.

While I have great respect for those who taught me the science and art of medicine, it took me twenty years to pay off the six-figure debt I racked up while learning it. That's about all the money my med-school professors are getting from me, and if their kids want to become doctors, I'd recommend a 529 plan rather than counting on my teaching them for free. Also, I'm not clear on whether this means I can justifiably charge their daughters tuition, or are their daughters forbidden from practicing medicine altogether according to this Oath?

I will apply dietetic measures for the benefit of the sick according to my ability and judgment; I will keep them from harm and injustice.

Keeping anyone from harm and injustice always sounds pretty reasonable to me. This correlates with another dictum of medicine: Primum, non nocere, or "First, do no harm." While I agree with the sentiment, I may define doing harm differently than many other doctors.

I will neither give a deadly drug to anybody if asked for it, nor will I make a suggestion to this effect.

Sorry, but after seeing my share of patients dying with indescribable suffering, I refuse to promise this to anyone. The profession of medicine should use its collective knowledge and compassion to relieve suffering, not propagate it and inflict it on those who are most vulnerable.

Similarly, I will not give a woman a pessary to cause an abortion.

I'm an ER doc. I don't perform abortions. If I did, however, I suppose I would agree that a pessary is not the best way to go about it, but I defer to my colleagues in OB/GYN.

Whatever houses I may visit, I will come for the benefit of the sick, remaining free of all intentional injustice, of all mischief and in particular of sexual relations with both female and male persons, be they free or slaves.

I understand why I shouldn't have sex with my free male or female patients, but not even the slaves? This passage illustrates the problem with any aged document, including those that are relatively much newer than the Hippocratic Oath, such as the U.S. Constitution. While the Constitution was designed to be a living document, it seems to be living in much the same condition as many of the nursing home patients we see in the ER every day. I'm not saying the Constitution has a sodium of 170 and renal failure because no one gives it water, or that it developed pneumonia after falling out of its bed in the Smithsonian and no one found it for 16 hours. Both of those things are not uncommon occurrences in nursing home patients, by the way.

What I mean is that the Constitution might technically be alive but isn't really enjoying the quality of life it envisioned at a younger age. I don't blame the Founding Fathers. I have no doubt they would have updated the Constitution periodically so that ~~Negroes~~ ~~coloreds~~ ~~Afro-Americans~~ ~~Blacks~~ African Americans would count as three-fifths of a person.

What I may see or hear in the course of the treatment or even outside of the treatment in regard to the life of men, which on no account one must spread abroad, I will keep to myself holding such things shameful to be spoken about.
Who put the HIPAA in Hippocrates?

If I fulfill this oath and do not violate it, it may be granted to me to enjoy life and art, being honored with fame among all men for all time to come.
Being honored with fame among all men for all time to come? Now *that* sounds impressive! Sign me up.

If I transgress it and swear falsely, may the opposite be my lot.
Never mind. The risk-to-benefit ratio just isn't there.

I understand that the part about being forced by the U.S. government to provide our services free of charge thanks to an unfunded government mandate was lost in the original translation from Greek. I'm afraid that without it, though, the Hippocratic Oath just isn't a document I can get behind.

Do I hear a second?

CHAPTER TWELVE

Finding the Lord in Room 3B

The ER is a place with a lot going on, theologically speaking.

For starters, about every six months an ambulance rolls in with a mentally ill man who claims to be Jesus. You've undoubtedly heard of "delusions of grandeur." I've always found it interesting that the mentally ill always have to be the head honcho, the top banana—usually God, Jesus, or Satan. No one ever claims to be John the Baptist or Judas or a Pope from the 16th Century. Nope—they're always in a lead role.

As you'd expect, He does tend to make a grand entrance, usually amidst the utter chaos of a busy shift. It's tough to recognize Him at first, since His head is often covered with a spit mask. Sadly, the Lord often tries to bite or spit at those trying to help Him. I'd always been taught that Jesus was a man of great restraint. No kidding: 4-point restraints, to be exact, usually made from leather.

He does actually look like the image most of us think of—a bit disheveled, not fully clothed, with long hair. And no wonder He wanted people to wash His feet; I often wish someone would.

Jesus preaches a lot, as you would expect, I guess. He's constantly yapping that "the end is near" or that the man in the gurney next to Him is the devil, which I find to be strangely coincidental. Once in a while, he tries to cast out the demon by screaming something along the lines of, "I'm gonna fucking kill you, man!" Jesus can be such a potty mouth.

I've also heard Jesus use the term "faggot" rather harshly and derogatorily. I never wanted to believe that Jesus was actually as homophobic as so many of His followers, but maybe it's true. I still find it disheartening.

As you might expect, Jesus possesses superhuman strength, particularly when jacked up on PCP or meth. I've wondered if Jesus drinks only Budweiser; the King of Beers for the King of Jews.

I must admit, it always disappoints me when Jesus' urine drug screen is positive. Jesus definitely loves Him some "burning bush."

I've been tempted to push a large rock in front of Jesus' room and check back in three days to see if He's still there. Instead, I usually just hydrate Him, give Him some Ativan, let His buzz wear off, remove the occasional rectal foreign body, and have the social worker see Him. After all, who should know better that the Lord helps those who help themselves?

I once cared for a woman who told me she was nine months pregnant. When I asked if she had picked out a name, she said, "It's the Messiah."

"That's going to be a hard one to live up to, isn't it?" I inquired curiously.

"He *is* the Messiah," she offered.

While my initial reaction was to blow this off, I started to think, "What if she was telling the truth?" If so, the only logical thing to do would be to marry her. Come on, you gotta admit, it would be pretty cool to be stepfather to the Son of God. You could put that on a resume or something, couldn't you?

As I thought it through, however, I realized that ultimately it would only lead to problems down the road.

When the Second Coming becomes a rebellious teenager, would I really want to be the stepfather? I can picture it now. Junior, as you call Him, sneaks in the door at 3 a.m. You smell the booze on Him and confront Him.

"What have you been drinking?"

"Water," He says with His usual cocky tone.

You glare at Him until He says, "Well, it *was* water!"

You both start arguing until He finally says it.

"You're not my real dad! My real dad invented the universe!"

Then you get defensive and say something like "Yeah, well, I've actually slept with your mom."

Things only go downhill from there, until you say something you might regret for... well... eternity.

"I can't wait until Easter!"

My mind eventually came back around to the fact that the woman who claimed to be nine months pregnant with the Messiah wasn't pregnant at all, rather she needed a psych consult.

I think some of God's followers should learn a thing or two from medicine. In a hospital, doctors are discouraged from giving "verbal orders." If I ask a nurse to do something, they might forget, hear it wrong, or remember it incorrectly, and the potential confusion could result in patient harm. We are told to write the order down whenever possible so that everyone can verify that the order is correct and appropriate for the patient.

Likewise, the same principle should apply to verbal orders from God. When God tells someone to drown all their children, or to set his wife on fire while she sleeps, maybe they should demand to see an order from God in writing before carrying it out. It would solve a lot of problems.

These anecdotes, while based on actual encounters, are obviously told tongue-in cheek, with no intent to offend anyone's religious beliefs. While I'm not a believer myself, I've been tempted to give a shout out in case anyone may be listening during a pediatric resuscitation or imminent airway disaster. In medicine, a smart doctor will take all the help they can get.

Amen.

CHAPTER THIRTEEN

The Most Important Trait in Medicine

Originally published on Doximity Op-Med, November 13, 2018

We've all dealt with the cocky consultant with his condescending tone and wondered why someone who seems to have no interest in actually helping people went into medicine. Personality disorders aside, what I find most perplexing is how anyone who has been practicing medicine for any length of time could possibly maintain such unrestrained arrogance.

Admittedly, I was more full of myself as a younger doctor and man. I can't say exactly when I learned perhaps the most important trait of being a doctor: humility. I can, however, recount numerous times when I've been humbled in medicine, which I suppose over time have instilled a sense of humility into my practice and my personality.

One of these "character-building" episodes most prominent in my memory was the first time I put in a central line as an intern. As a medical student, I had been fortunate to do a fair number of procedures, including central lines. I placed several smoothly enough to foolishly think I was a natural.

Fast forward to internship, when my senior resident asked me and one of my classmates, Bill, if we had ever put in a central line. I said "Yes, several." Bill had never done one.

"Great," the senior resident said. "Take Bill with you and show him how to do one, will you?"

The notion that I would be teaching my fellow intern only reinforced my self-assuredness. I gathered the equipment, explaining "my approach" to the procedure to Bill, based on my weeks of experience, and we went to the patient's bedside. The patient, Mr. J, was an elderly man with advanced dementia and severe kyphosis whose shoulders were rounded forward and inward. I was to place a subclavian line. I couldn't get his shoulders into a more natural position and knew that the angle of insertion wasn't going to be "what I was used to," as if I was now some sort of expert. This wasn't the time for self-doubt, however. It was the time to show Bill who was who in our intern class.

Long story short, after making a pin cushion out of Mr. J for a half hour, the only blood I had to show for it was the hematoma I'd caused. After seeing me flail and fail miserably, the shoe was clearly on the other foot, with Bill undoubtedly thinking to himself, "Yes, I guess we know who's who now, don't we?" Reticent to abandon my efforts, I tried the other side before finally surrendering long after a reasonable number of attempts had passed.

The best part? After botching my attempt to impress Bill and my senior resident, as well as further inflate my ego, I failed to get access and managed to drop Mr. J's lung in the process. That's right—my very first attempt at a central line as an ER resident resulted in an iatrogenic pneumothorax. To top it off, the senior resident let Bill put in the chest tube, something I had never done.

Simply put, it was a karmic smackdown of epic proportions. It actually personified karma, as if karma had read my mind, started shaking its head and chuckling, then sat me down and said, "*I've got something for you.*"

Mind you, this wasn't the first dumb thing I'd ever done. There was the time in med school on my neurology rotation when I was testing sensation in the feet of a patient with multiple sclerosis. I didn't have a safety pin, so I brilliantly improvised with a hypodermic needle I pulled out of the cabinet in the patient's room (this was back in the day, before a retinal scan and chain of custody form were required to obtain vital medical supplies such as needles, or Hemoccult developer). I meticulously tested about ten spots on each foot, obliviously recording each jolted response of "Sharp!"

Seconds later I looked down in horror at the ten drops of blood on the patient's feet. I attempted to coolly act as though this was just part of the process as I quickly wiped off the blood. Any illusion I had that the patient was none the wiser was erased when, during attending rounds, he proclaimed, "Don't worry, Reggie. The bleeding stopped."

Fortunately, my attending had no idea what the patient could have been referring to, since bloodletting wasn't big in neurology. Yes, I was a real "medical MacGyver," with one subtle difference between us: MacGyver wasn't an idiot.

My misguided lung biopsy on Mr. J was also far from the last failure I've experienced in medicine, but here's the thing: I've had a lot of successes, too. Over the course of my career, I've been privileged to play a role in some of the most poignant, resilient and tragic moments in patients' lives. I've been devastated and elated. Right and wrong. Laser-focused and distracted. Compassionate and burned-out. Human.

I've never lost sight of the fact that while expansive knowledge and refined technical skills are what we all aspire to, sometimes a little luck goes a long way. I've been the heroic "second doctor" to swoop in and save the day when a colleague couldn't get an LP or reduce a joint. I've also learned not to be afraid to ask for help when things aren't going my way, or the patient's, and to let one of my friends come to the rescue without permanently damaging my sense of self-worth. I'm grateful for all the times I've nailed the procedure or stumbled upon the correct diagnosis without ever fully understanding how.

Medicine is a humbling profession, and anyone who has worked in a difficult environment with lives on the line must know that. If you don't, you just haven't been paying attention.

CHAPTER FOURTEEN

I Didn't Mean to Insult You

If there's one attribute that sets ER doctors apart from most other physicians, it's having a finely tuned bullshit meter. Patients routinely lie about things big and small. It's why we always check a pregnancy test on a young woman with abdominal pain no matter how much she insists that she can't possibly be pregnant. It's why we get urine drug screens on patients who claim they don't use drugs. It's comical that some of these patients think *we're* the ones who are clueless. Trust me, if you think you're pulling one over on us, I can almost guarantee we're on to you.

Chief complaint: Confusion

A 37-year-old woman reeking of alcohol came in with her boyfriend. She'd told her boyfriend, however, that she hadn't had anything to drink. He was quite concerned about her symptoms. He said her speech had become slurred and she couldn't walk straight. He also thought she seemed confused. He actually said the words, "It's almost like she's intoxicated, but I know that's not it."

A BAL (blood alcohol level) of 0.28 begged to differ (0.08 is the legal limit to drive). I told the guy that she was drunk, and in fact was over three times the legal limit to drive. She still tried to keep up the charade, acting innocent as she said with a straight face, "What would account for that?"

I stated emphatically, "Drinking."

Chief complaint: Overdose

At about 0320 one night (morning?) a guy called the nursing hotline to say "My girlfriend OD'd on a lot of shit, man! We'll be there in two minutes! Make sure someone is waiting for us!"

Working in the ER, it's not uncommon for someone to do a quick drop-off in front of the ambulance doors in the middle of the night, often for someone who's not breathing because of a heroin overdose. They don't want to answer questions or get themselves in legal trouble, but they don't want their buddy to die, either, so they get them as far as the front door.

We watched the parking lot camera, and sure enough, about two minutes later a car came screeching to a stop in front of the ambulance entrance and a tall, young man got out and ran around to the other side of the car. He frantically opened the front passenger door and scooped up his girlfriend before sprinting toward the ambulance entrance carrying a 19-year-old girl who appeared to be awake and alert. Already it seemed a bit anti-climactic; usually the person dropped off is blue, not breathing, and you have to check a pulse to see if you need to start CPR. She looked remarkably stable from a distance.

As she was carried to a gurney, I began asking questions.

"What did you take?

He answered for her. "She shot up some heroin."

Well-known to the lay public due to the opioid epidemic, which is currently a far bigger problem than it was at that time, you may have heard about naloxone, or Narcan, which is an antidote for an opioid overdose. I wasn't sure she'd need it, as she was breathing and able to talk, so I asked a follow-up question.

"Did you take anything else?"

The patient responded. "I did a couple lines of coke."

"Anything else?" I asked.

Her boyfriend this time: "She also took some OxyContin."

OxyContin is a powerful opioid as well, and is abused several different ways, so I asked how she had used it.

Her boyfriend said, "She took some pills."

She added, "I shot some of it too. And I snorted some."

More just because it's what you do—keep asking questions until you get a "No," I kept going.

"Anything else?"

They both replied, "We did some E earlier." "E" meant ecstasy, a stimulant. It was beginning to make sense why she wasn't comatose. She had enough uppers and downers in her to counteract many of the side effects of the other.

They both also admitted to smoking marijuana.

I had one last question.

"Have you had anything to drink?"

They both looked at me as if completely offended, and snapped back at me in disgust, "We don't drink!"

I once saw a meth addict who told me he ate it, snorted it, smoked it and injected it, all on the same day. I'm not sure if that reflects serious motivation or major indecision.

I also once saw a 65-year-old meth user. I thought to myself, "When most people look forward to using their Grandma's crystal, they're referring to the Waterford."

You might think all the lying and trying to manipulate us is insulting. It's actually more amusing than anything. When you show up in the ER with track marks all over your body and tell me you don't inject drugs but think you were "bitten by a spider," my advice is to stop sharing spiders.

It is disturbing, though, when you refuse to take responsibility for your actions, especially when those actions harm your children. I once was taking a history from a mother about her young daughter, and when I asked if she had any medical problems, her mother offered, "She was born positive for meth." She was "born positive?" Was it immaculate injection? I know it must be hard as a mother to say, "I was a meth addict during my entire pregnancy."

Sometimes you can use the information you're given to your advantage.

Chief complaint: "I think there might be something in my ass."

A 44-year-old male presented to the ER high as a kite on crack: jittery, anxious, and sweating buckets. He was lying flat on his stomach and wouldn't even roll over to talk to me. Then he told me why he was there. He said he *thought* there was something *in his ass*—and this is the part that got me—but he *wasn't sure*. Seriously, has that ever happened to you? Have you ever wondered, "Is there something in my ass right now? I really can't tell."

I noticed he was wearing jeans, so I asked him how that could have happened. He said he got "pretty messed up," and he thought someone may have taken his pants down and inserted something into his ass *without him noticing*.

Dear Reader, have you *ever* been that messed up? I've *always* been able to tell when there's something in my ass. That's why I got *out* of the Army. Ba-dum-bum.

This guy wasn't sure, though.

He's lying there, face down on the table. I figure I have to do a rectal exam on this guy: yes, that's the glamorous part of the job they don't show on TV.

All of the sudden he started thrashing around and freaking out.

"What's wrong?" I asked.

In a classic ER moment, his voice wavered as he nervously whispered, "I think I can feel it moving!"

I have to admit, I was getting a little freaked out myself at that point. I reacted like the trained medical professional that I was, jumping quickly back from the bed. I mean, if I do a rectal exam on this guy, am I going to get bitten?

Then he told me he wanted an x-ray to see what it was. At that point it was pretty clear that this was one jacked-up dude, and there was (probably) nothing in his ass. I did the x-ray just to pacify him, though, and of course it didn't show anything.

Then I got what I thought was a brilliant idea. I marched into his room and told him the straight-up, God's-honest truth.

"Dude, you were right! I can't tell what it is, but as God is my witness, I haven't seen that many teeth since Shark Week on the Discovery Channel!"

Years of education to become an emergency physician: 24.

Total debt acquired in becoming an emergency physician: $200,000.

Look on a patient's face after telling him there is something with a lot of teeth in his ass: priceless.

I continued, "It looks like it's sleeping, so whatever you do, you need to lay here *very* still and *very* quietly." I told him I would give him something to help sedate the creature. I ordered some lorazepam (Ativan) for him, a benzodiazepine related to Valium, which we give so frequently in the ER it is referred to as "Vitamin A."

To seal the deal in convincing him I was taking this seriously, I told him I was going to try to coax it out, so I taped a piece of cheese to his ass. OK, I didn't actually do this part, but I told my attending physician I was going to do it just to make him laugh. It is somewhat perverse that it's OK to use drugs to the point that you can't tell whether or not you have an animal in your ass, but my taping cheese to his ass would have crossed a line?

That's how I got a jacked-up crack user to lay very politely and quietly in our ER. He eventually fell asleep and stayed that way for the next ten hours. I remain convinced it was at that moment, during the second week of my first year of residency, that I was officially considered the front-runner to become Chief Resident.

CHAPTER FIFTEEN

The Handprint

Jane was 41 on the day she came to the ER feeling short of breath. Her fate was sealed before that day arrived; she had stage IV lung cancer with metastases to her bones and brain. Her disease had progressed to the point that her oncologist had spoken to her about hospice care, but Jane had a few more things she wanted to do before her time was up. She traveled to see family over Thanksgiving weekend. She was planning to spend what she knew would be her last Christmas with loved ones.

The day before Thanksgiving she had a scant amount of hemoptysis, meaning she coughed up small amounts of blood. This happened a few times over the weekend as well. She figured she'd follow up with her oncologist after the holiday when she returned home, but she became short of breath and was experiencing slight chest pain, which prompted her to come to the ER.

Given her cancer, recent travel, hemoptysis and dyspnea (shortness of breath), combined with a chest x-ray that didn't show any pneumonia or other reason for her to feel short of breath, aside from her large, visible lung mass, from a medical standpoint the next step was pretty obvious: we needed to look for a pulmonary embolus, a blood clot in her lung, something which can be life-threatening and for which she was at very high risk.

A CT pulmonary angiogram was performed. The test involves injecting a bolus of intravenous contrast and timing it so that a high-resolution, high-speed CT can be done while the contrast is flowing through the blood vessels in the lungs to detect any obstruction to blood flow caused by a clot. Fortunately, Jane's CT pulmonary angiogram was negative. She didn't have a pulmonary embolus, though her left upper lung mass, the cancer that ravaged her body, had increased in size and was wrapped around an artery in her chest.

Her other testing also being fairly unremarkable, I spoke to her oncologist about next steps. We agreed that she should follow up in a day or two, at which time her oncologist would again raise the issue of hospice, as her time was growing short. I discussed all of her findings and the oncologist's recommendations with Jane, and she and her fiancé felt comfortable going home.

I had just hit "Print" on her discharge instructions when her fiancé came out to the desk where I was sitting to tell me she had just coughed up more blood. I went to go look for myself.

I walked into the room to see Jane hunched over the kick bucket her fiancé had grabbed off the floor. She was trying to cough but looked as though she was having trouble doing so. Once she did, she brought up an alarming amount of blood at once. I had seen patients vomit that much blood before, but this was coming from her lung, not her stomach. When coming from the stomach, what you often see is blood mixed with a fair amount of digestive fluids so that the amount of bleeding looks exaggerated. Coming from Jane's lung, this was all blood.

When I was close enough to see inside the shiny silver trash receptacle, I visualized what I estimated to be a liter and a half of blood. After gasping to take another deep breath, she again tried to cough, but the only thing that came out was another huge gush of blood.

She looked up at me with pleading eyes and mouthed the words "Help me," though no sound came out. She grabbed my shirt as if begging. Blood kept flowing out of her mouth. Jane looked terrified. So did her fiancé. So did I, I'm sure.

Perhaps the most critical skill in emergency medicine is being able to distinguish which patients are truly ill from those who are not; what we refer to as "sick" or "not sick." When *we* say sick, we don't mean you look like you have a cold. We mean we are worried about you. You potentially have a dangerous or even life-threatening illness or injury.

In those split seconds, I knew that Jane wasn't just sick. I knew she would be dead in the next minute, maybe two.

Jane hadn't yet filled out advanced directives or made any specific wishes known. That meant she was a "full code," which usually implies that we would do everything we possibly could to try to resuscitate her. Now, though, no one was going to save her. Jane was exsanguinating and asphyxiating simultaneously— bleeding to death and suffocating at the same time. And there was nothing I could do to stop it.

I looked into her fiancé's eyes and told him, "I'm sorry. She's dying, and there is nothing I can do to stop it. This is the end." I didn't know what else to say, but I didn't need to explain any more. He understood.

Jane became very pale and diaphoretic (sweaty) as she retched twice more, each time bringing up another significant quantity of blood. As she continued to lean over the wastebasket, I felt her slump forward, become heavy and lifeless, and I knew that she was now unconscious. Blood continued to ooze from her mouth, a sight I didn't think her husband-to-be needed to see, so I did my best to coolly support her weight with one hand until blood stopped streaming into the bucket.

As I gently laid her back, I quickly wiped the blood from her face. Jane was dead.

I did my best to console her fiancé and explained that her cancer had likely eroded through the wall of the large blood vessel it had been surrounding. There was nothing anybody could have done about it. He was aware that her time had been running out, making the fact that she died unsurprising, but to watch it happen like that, right in front of him, was traumatic.

I'd seen people bleed to death from gunshot wounds and from GI (gastrointestinal) bleeding. I'd never seen anyone die like that, though: scared, silently begging for help, unable to breathe while bleeding to death. It shook me.

After leaving Jane's side, I went to the bathroom to splash some water on my face and process what I had just witnessed. I ran the water until it was as cold as I could get it, then cupped my hands under the faucet, raising them to douse my face, which felt almost hot to the touch. I took some deep breaths, grabbed some paper towel, and began to dry my face.

I stood up straight and looked into the mirror when I saw it: Jane's bloody handprint right in the center of my pressed white dress shirt. I began to sob.

I took the next few minutes to do something we so rarely allow ourselves to do in medicine: grieve. I eventually regained my composure. I did my best to wash the blood out of my shirt, buttoned my lab coat in an attempt to conceal the spot, and returned to my workstation. Since I was only about halfway through my shift, I signed up for my next patient, a young boy with a dog bite. After suffering the emotional trauma of holding a fellow traveler upright as she took her last breath, a few minutes later I did my best to give the rest of my patients on that shift the same attention and care that I had given Jane.

It helped to talk to my colleagues about it. They all get it. Emergency physicians spend countless hours reading and studying, developing skills, perfecting techniques, mastering procedures and practicing emergency medicine so that we can save a life when the time comes. We rehearse nightmarish scenarios, knowing that one day we might experience them. We spend hours in labs learning to manage difficult airways or obtain IV access. We know that our knowledge and skills may determine whether a patient might live or die. It is an extraordinary responsibility, yet it's why we chose this profession.

It isn't natural to stand by and do nothing in those moments, yet sometimes that is exactly what we should do. Sometimes the kindest act we can perform is to assure a loved one that they did everything they could, and perhaps to wipe the blood from a face and absorb as much of the trauma as you can in order to save them from it.

One of the privileges of emergency medicine is sharing the most poignant and profound of human experiences with strangers who imprint indelible memories that become part of your own journey through life. You remember the look on her face; the pleading in her eyes; watching her take her last breath. You never forget the handprint.

CHAPTER SIXTEEN

Fight Club and Gurney Races

Nothing breaks up the monotony of a night shift like a BAL (blood alcohol level) pool on some drunk asshole who is puking or shitting on himself, swearing at the top of his lungs, and who either fell down and broke his face or drove his pickup over a family of five. To pass the time, one of the nurses starts a pool, collecting money from each participant. For your cash you get to guess how high his BAL is, and whoever is closest gets the cash.

When you're new to the ER you tend to guess low...way low. You consider the fact that the legal limit to drive is 0.08. You figure this guy is clearly impaired, but he's still talking (swearing) and walking (stumbling over to the corner to take a leak on the wall), so his BAL must be more like twice that, so you write down "0.15". You're feeling good about it until his level comes back from the lab at 0.42. "How is that possible?" you ask yourself. "I'd be in a coma." One of the nurses wins the pool. A nurse always does.

The sheer number of ER visits related to drug, alcohol, and mental health problems is staggering. I recall a night shift during which I had nine patients in the department at 3 a.m. who were all drunk.

At the time, our largest room had five gurneys separated only by curtains. Needless to say, you might not have been able to *see* what's going on "next door," but you could certainly *hear* it. This room was filled with four drunk patients and a fifth patient who was an LOL (little old lady) with a hip fracture. Three of the drunks were there after having been involved in fights. Two had split lips that needed to be sutured, one had two teeth knocked out, and the fourth had fallen down and hit his head.

The four young men proceeded to swap war stories about their various bar fights.

"Man, I punched that fucker right in the face!"

"Man, I would have killed that mother fucker!"

"Fuck yeah, dude! I fucking hate that fuck!"

We moved the LOL to another room.

In her place a fifth drunk arrived, which seemed to give the room a sense of unity in purpose.

Two of the other drunks in the department at the time had been driving, one of whom had caused an accident. Amazingly, no one was injured in the other vehicle. Usually the drunk walks away without a scratch while law enforcement is scrounging around for dental records to identify the innocent occupants of the other vehicle. This is a part of emergency medicine I've always struggled with, knowing that this asshole could have killed someone I love, yet I'm supposed to treat him with respect and compassion? Hard to do at times. Especially when the guy is wearing an electronic ankle bracelet, proving he's not one to follow the rules anyway. Ironically, he also sported an "Alcoholics Anonymous" tattoo. I guess the tattoo doesn't actually prevent alcohol from getting into your bloodstream.

The night dragged on forever, as night shifts usually do.

In a moment of levity, as I was working in close proximity, a patient said to me, "You have really pretty eyes."

It was one of the drunk guys. I was putting stitches in his busted lip. I guess you just have to take a compliment where you can get one. "Thanks," I responded.

As I continued working, I couldn't help but think of the movie Fight Club, and how I'd propose my own rules for the ER.

The first rule of Fight Club is you don't talk about Fight Club.

The second rule of Fight Club is if you're smashed off your ass, you might lose at Fight Club.

The third rule of Fight Club is if you lose at Fight Club, don't bring your dumb ass to the ER.

Two of the drunks had blowout fractures, meaning the bone that forms the floor of the orbit, which is basically what your eye rests on, was broken. Four of them required complex laceration repairs. After this barrage of drunks, near the end of my shift, however, the monotony was broken up nicely by an 18-year-old female who awoke with some cramping and vaginal bleeding.

Despite the fact that the patient weighed no more than 110 pounds, the basketball-sized protrusion with stretch marks on it that "got really painful every two or three minutes" failed to provide a clue to this girl that she was, in fact, pregnant and about to deliver any minute.

When I asked about her pregnancy, which could not have been more obvious, she stated, while panting through a contraction, "I'm not pregnant."

The hair-covered scalp beginning to protrude from her vagina begged otherwise.

Thus began the gurney race down to Labor & Delivery for the girl who couldn't figure out what in the world was happening to her this morning since she knew she wasn't pregnant.

Her mother, who I quickly deduced wasn't exactly a NASA engineer herself, told me everything I needed to know when she said, "Oh! This must have happened before her boyfriend went to prison."

CHAPTER SEVENTEEN

Three Useful Tips

Now, for the public service portion of the book, I will address some myths I frequently hear in the ER.

1. "My wound won't get infected because it bled a lot."

Quantity of bleeding has little to do with how clean a wound is. What's important is how much dirt gets into the wound. Bleeding a lot after cutting yourself on rusty metal covered in pig feces is not good. You need to clean the wound out thoroughly.

As an example of the importance of being able to clean a wound, cat bites get infected about 90% of the time. Why? Because the small puncture wounds don't allow you to clean the wound out. You're essentially just wiping the skin off. Bacteria are inoculated into the subcutaneous tissue where they can't be flushed out because the puncture wounds from the cat's teeth are so tiny.

Dog bites get infected about 25% of the time because a dog's teeth cause bigger holes. The larger wounds bleed more but provide an opening to be able to flush out the bacteria. Blood is actually an excellent medium in which bacteria can grow. It's a myth that bleeding a lot helps prevent infection. Clean the wound.

2. "A high fever will fry my child's brain."

No, it won't. Fever from a cold or ear infection is not dangerous, no matter how high it gets. It is true that extremely high body temperature can be part of life-threatening conditions such as heat stroke, malignant hyperthermia, neuroleptic malignant syndrome, and drug overdoses such as cocaine, ecstasy, or methamphetamines.

More often, though, fever is part of your body's response to fighting an infection. Having said that, fever can induce febrile seizures, and it's hard for me to tell parents not to worry about their child having a seizure. When it happens, it's terrifying. If your child has a febrile seizure, however, it doesn't mean they will have epilepsy or be prone to seizures later in life.

The notion that high fever will cause brain damage didn't appear out of thin air. In the 1970s, children with viral illnesses, especially chicken pox, who were given aspirin occasionally developed Reye Syndrome, which did in fact result in permanent brain damage or death in some cases. This is probably why fever became associated with brain damage, but rest assured that fever from a routine childhood illness will not "fry your child's brain."

Like many lessons in human history, not giving children aspirin was learned the hard way. I am old enough to remember baby aspirin from those days. They were orange-flavored and tasted like candy. Aspirin is lethal in large quantities. Leaving a bottle of candy-flavored pills lying around that could induce Reye syndrome or salicylate toxicity was so 1970s!

3. "My nosebleed won't stop even though I put ice on my neck and tilted my head back."

A semester-long first aid course should be required of every high school student. The principle of how to stop bleeding is something every citizen should understand. Tragically, because of the number of mass shootings and terrorist attacks around the world, we have probably all become more familiar with some level of understanding of how to stop bleeding.

The primary method is simple: direct pressure. Most nosebleeds occur in the front of the nose, and pinching the nostrils together firmly will stop most nosebleeds. I've seen patients walk into triage with their heads tilted back and blood pouring all over their shirts and the floor. "I can't get the bleeding to stop!" they exclaim.

Wad up a small piece of toilet paper and gently twist it into the nostril that is bleeding, then pinch your nostrils together. It may take some time, but if you hold firm pressure long enough, the bleeding should stop. If you have a lot of blood running down the back of your throat, or if you take blood thinners of any kind or are older, you should go to an ER to be evaluated. If you are young, healthy, and don't take any blood thinners, nosebleeds are rarely problematic. Hold pressure until it stops, and don't worry about nosebleeds unless they become frequent or can't be controlled this way.

CHAPTER EIGHTEEN

I Need a Nurse in CT STAT

Chief complaint: "Abdominal pain"

A 39-year-old man presents at 0600 by ambulance complaining of intense abdominal cramps since midnight. He thought maybe he'd eaten something bad. He had nausea but no vomiting, diarrhea, fever, chills, and had no blood in his stool.

His exam didn't elicit any specific tenderness in any part of his belly that helped narrow down the list of potential causes of his pain. I ordered some pain medication and initiated the usual belly labs: CBC (complete blood count), LFTs (liver function tests), Chem-8 (basic metabolic panel) and a lipase. They screen for infection, bleeding, pancreatitis, liver problems, gallbladder problems, kidney function, diabetes, acid-base disturbances and electrolyte imbalances, among others.

His white blood cell count was a little above normal, and given his degree of pain, I wanted to obtain imaging in the form of a CT scan to see if we could find the cause of his pain.

My shift was ending at 0700. By the time his labs were back and I ordered his CT, my relief was there. I handed the patient off to the oncoming physician, my friend Andy, who would evaluate his CT result and *dispo* the patient accordingly (short for disposition—figuring out whether the patient could go home or needed to stay in the hospital).

Earlier in my shift I had been talking to Rob, one of our excellent ER nurses, as we were both tech-geeks and liked to discuss the latest gadgets and gizmos. As I was walking out the door, Rob stopped me to asked me if I had looked at the watch we discussed. I turned around and walked about six feet back to the counter next to Rob's workstation, tired and wanting to go home to sleep, but always happy to talk to Rob about electronics or anything else. About 30 seconds later I heard yelling from down the hall.

"I need a nurse in CT STAT!"

Knowing it was my abdominal pain patient who was in the CT scanner, I followed several staff members running down the hall to investigate.

As I entered the radiology suite, the patient appeared to be having a seizure. He was lifting his head up off the gurney and his arms were pulled up to his chest and shaking rhythmically. His face was purple due to the fact that oxygen wasn't getting to his head and neck because the intense muscle contraction was preventing him from breathing normally.

We proceeded to roll him back down the hallway into our resuscitation room. My mind starting racing through a differential diagnosis, a list of possible causes, that would explain what would cause severe abdominal pain *and* a seizure.

His body relaxed as the seizure seemed to subside. As the nurses hooked him up to monitors, I checked for a pulse, and could not find one. His cardiac monitor provided the reason: he was in v-fib, ventricular fibrillation. Defibrillator pads were immediately placed on his chest.

"Everyone stand clear!" I said firmly. I pushed the red button with the lightning bolt on it, and his body heaved upward as the defibrillator delivered 200 joules of biphasic energy through his chest.

He was no longer in v-fib, but he still didn't have a pulse, and the disorganized, sporadic electrical impulses displayed on the screen indicated he was still dead.

"Start compressions," I ordered next, though I didn't need to—ER staff know exactly what to do in such a crisis.

Andy, to whom I had just turned the patient over, had already begun assembling equipment to intubate the patient. As it turned out, we were just getting started.

Andy expertly slid the clear polyvinylchloride tube past the dead man's vocal cords into his trachea as our ER techs took turns doing superb chest compressions. I stood next to the man's right hip with my right index and middle fingers over his femoral artery. This allowed me to feel the pulse that traveled under my fingers with each chest compression. Periodically I would tell the tech "Hold CPR" so that I could check to see if the patient had regained a pulse (ROSC—return of spontaneous circulation, as you may recall).

As our team made every effort, I realized that the odds were against us as the minutes passed without any change in the patient's rhythm. For a short period of time, his rhythm deteriorated to asystole, or what is referred to as "flatline"—no electrical activity whatsoever—which was even worse.

We administered epinephrine and amiodarone in repeated doses to try to stimulate his heart and regulate its rhythm. No effect.

Almost forty minutes into the code, with no sign of improvement, it was about time to call it—to stop our efforts and pronounce him dead. As I usually do in similar circumstances, I asked the team if anyone had any other ideas or any concerns over stopping our efforts. Yes, I'm the ER doctor, ultimately responsible for such things, but being part of a patient's death is a profound experience that takes a toll on the entire team. For a 96-year-old from a nursing home whose existence was composed primarily of suffering, pronouncing death makes sense to everyone; but for a previously healthy 39-year-old who came in just an hour before, talking and complaining of abdominal pain, I wanted to check with all the staff to be sure.

We were all on the same page. I therefore asked the tech to pause chest compressions one more time for a final pulse check. When a patient is in asystole, the first course of action is to check a second lead. The last thing you want to do is to pronounce a patient dead only to find out they were very much alive, but that a monitoring lead had popped off during CPR. Anticipating seeing asystole and ready to ask to check a second lead, I was surprised to see what appeared to be a fairly organized electrical impulse on the monitor. This was followed by another, then another, and actually looked like a decent electrical rhythm. Most importantly, my fingers could feel a pulse!

Weak at first, his pulse quickly gained strength to the point that we were able to obtain an adequate blood pressure. An ECG revealed the true nature of his problem: he was having a heart attack! The patient clearly didn't think he was having a heart attack, or he wouldn't have stayed home for six hours with the pain. The paramedics didn't suspect a heart attack, or they would have done an ECG themselves and transported him to an ER in a hospital that contained a cath lab. I hadn't pursued it, either, given his age, good health and generalized abdominal pain rather than epigastric pain which is more often associated with potential heart problems.

The patient was alive, but after forty minutes of CPR and resuscitation, the real question was whether we had done him any favors. Perhaps a fate worse than death is suffering permanent neurologic disability, having caregivers wipe the drool from your chin for the rest of your days.

I followed his hospital course day by day. For the first 24 hours he was "cooled." Therapeutic hypothermia, cooling the body's core temperature to around 32 degrees Celsius, or about 90 Fahrenheit, has been proven to result in improved neurologic outcome after a v-fib cardiac arrest. That doesn't mean *everyone* does better, of course, only that you have a better chance of waking up with something resembling an intact melon than you would without cooling.

He survived the 24-hour cooling period, but the post-resuscitation complications came fast and furious. The lack of perfusion (blood flow) to his kidneys resulted in renal failure leading to dialysis (a different form of dialysis called CRRT, actually, because he was too sick to tolerate dialysis). An infusion of a vasopressor, a medication that constricts blood vessels in an effort to maintain enough blood pressure to sustain life, infiltrated (leaked) out of the vein into the surrounding tissue. This caused some of the tissue to become necrotic (die), and the dead tissue had to be cut out and the skin grafted. He was encephalopathic, which is a fancy way of saying he was disoriented and confused. He didn't know if he was coming or going for weeks. He suffered nerve palsy in his leg, causing foot drop. The lack of blood flow to his intestines led to internal bleeding. He aspirated stomach contents into his lungs, causing infection and inflammation that required prolonged mechanical ventilation and intensive antibiotics.

Yet he survived, step by step, day by day, until I was amazed to read in his chart that he had been discharged home. He made it home! The odds were stacked heavily against him; patients with a down time of 40 minutes don't survive with a normally functioning brain very often.

He'd had some luck on his side that day. I'd been just a few feet from being out the door. What are the odds that Rob would stop me to ask about a watch, causing me to turn around and stay just a minute longer? And it wasn't just me: the fact that his cardiac arrest occurred during change of shift was fortuitous. Normally staffed with one physician, three nurses and one tech, change of shift meant we had two docs, six nurses and two techs. The techs and nurses were able to rotate, helping them maintain high quality chest compressions throughout the prolonged code. I was able to focus on the resuscitation while Andy secured his airway. We had twice the number of highly skilled ER nurses present to push meds, manage the defibrillator, watch the monitors, run some tests and everything else that needed to be done.

Our team saved his life! This solitary patient encounter at the end of a night shift, the last patient of my workday, was a microcosm of everything it means to be an emergency physician.

CHAPTER NINETEEN

Timing Is Everything

"It's better to be lucky than good." I don't know who first said it. I don't believe it's *better*—I'd rather be good, and being good is more directly in my control, but a little luck never hurt.

The timing of when a patient presents to the ER in the course of their disease process can make a world of difference. If you show up early on, your symptoms might be too non-specific, a term we use about a thousand times a day in the ER, to identify exactly what the problem is. If you wait longer than you should, maybe it's too late, and bad things happen.

Rare is the patient who presents to the ER within the precise few hours that their illness evolves from mild to severe: the patient who looks fine when they walk in the door, then crashes before they leave. Lots of patients present when they are fine and they stay that way, and a fair number present when they are critically ill, making them easy to spot. For the others, the luck of their timing might be what saved their lives, with help from those of us in the ER.

A 37-year-old woman presented in August with flu-like symptoms. When she walked in with her husband and children, she looked like she wasn't feeling well, but she wasn't what we call "sick." Her vital signs were OK except for fever and a rapid heart rate. She was positive for influenza A. It made sense given her flu-like symptoms, though was a bit unusual to see flu in August, having not seen any other flu cases yet that season.

During the relatively short time she was in the ER, she started to feel a little short of breath, so I ordered a chest x-ray that showed pneumonia on both sides. In combination with her other lab results and the fact that she kept feeling progressively worse, I determined that she needed to be admitted to the hospital, just to err on the side of caution. She continued a downward spiral, however, and I ended up intubating her and placing her on a ventilator. She ultimately spent a month in the hospital and nearly became one of tens of thousands of flu deaths each year. My aggressive intervention in the ER helped save her life, yet what if she had presented to me twelve, or six, or even three hours earlier? She would likely have been home again, not appearing ill enough to require hospitalization, and perhaps she would have stopped breathing in her family room because no one was there to intervene. Her coming to the ER precisely when she did might have made the difference between her living and dying.

This type of progression of disease keeps us up at night. A patient might look and feel well enough to go home. How do I know they will stay that way? How do I know they won't deteriorate and get sicker quickly at home? ER doctors make these kinds of judgement calls every day.

A 51-year-old man ran through the front door of the ER to the registration desk panicked that he was bleeding to death. Given the trail of bright red blood on the floor that followed him, I thought he might have been on to something. He was brought immediately back to the closest room. The blood spilling from his mouth all the way back to the room demanded my full attention.

He'd recently had a radical tonsillectomy for throat cancer and had just been upstairs to follow up with his otolaryngologist (ears, nose and throat doctor). Everything had looked good and he was on his way out the door when he suddenly began bleeding profusely.

I tried to look in his mouth, but he couldn't open it wide enough for me to see where the blood was coming from. I grabbed some gauze and shoved some in the back of his mouth on the side that looked like the general area of bleeding. I no sooner thought about what to do next when in sprinted his ENT from upstairs, Dr. Tristan Korman. Dr. Korman looked in his mouth and said to me, "He needs to be intubated right away."

"Say no more," I replied, and I directed the nurses as to the medications we would need and began gathering equipment. The nurse drew up 20 mg of etomidate, a sedative, and 150 mg of succinylcholine, a paralytic agent, as I opened the packaging on a laryngoscope, Mac-3 blade, endotracheal tube, stylet, 10 mL syringe, and carbon dioxide detector. As soon as an IV was established and medications were drawn up, I asked the nurse to push the meds. Once the patient was paralyzed, the ball was solely in my court. I inserted the laryngoscope blade into the right side of his mouth as I'd done many times before, sweeping his tongue to the left as I advanced the blade into his vallecula and lifted his epiglottis forward, revealing his vocal cords. I slid the ET tube past his vocal cords before withdrawing the laryngoscope and inflating the cuff on the tube with the 10 mL syringe. I attached the CO_2 colorimeter and confirmed tube placement while listening to his lungs, inspecting the tube for fogging, and watching the rise and fall of his chest. The ET tube was secured in place, and I turned the patient back over to Dr. Korman.

The patient's airway now protected and the patient paralyzed, Dr. Korman was able to open his mouth more widely and visualize the site of bleeding, but he couldn't stop it. He tried several techniques to no avail. Our ER had a limited blood supply at that moment because I was transfusing another patient with brisk GI bleeding. We called 911 to transfer the patient to our tertiary care center. Dr. Korman rode in the ambulance with his hand holding direct pressure inside the patient's mouth the entire time. The patient was transported directly to interventional radiology where embolization was performed to stabilize him.

The patient thought he was dying when he had arrived, and he was correct. It was quite serendipitous that his ENT was still in the building, able to respond immediately, and willing to accompany him in the ambulance. Had he started hemorrhaging at home a half hour later, he may have bled to death before making it to the ER. For some patients, *timing is everything.*

CHAPTER TWENTY

A Moment of Pride

Originally published in Emergency Physicians Monthly in 2004

During a recent flight I was reminded of what it truly means to be an emergency physician.

Let me first say that I'm not a big fan of flying. Why is it that the only thing that has room to shift during a flight is the luggage in the overhead compartment? It's no wonder that flights pose a risk of DVT: there isn't even enough room for a corpuscle to move through a vein! Anyway, I was wedged uncomfortably in my seat, trying to distract myself by listening to my iPod, when I opened my eyes and noticed there was a bit of commotion among the passengers. I heard a muffled announcement from a flight attendant, and removed my headphones to hear the announcement being repeated:

"If there is anyone on board with medical training, please identify yourself to a member of the flight crew."

I pried myself from my seat and walked sideways down the aisle to avoid every head that was turned to look toward the back of the plane, where a gentleman was clearly in distress.

Ashen, pale and diaphoretic, a 57-year-old man complained of epigastric discomfort and tightness in his chest. Also on board were a paramedic and a respiratory therapist. Not a bad combination to have, I thought to myself, if we needed to run a code.

As I first approached the man, he looked quite concerned, which was understandable. After all, there I was in my scarlet and gray 'Ohio State 2002 National Champions' T-shirt, while he wore the purple and gold of the University of Washington Huskies, a team my beloved Buckeyes had trounced just one day prior. "Perfect! I'm dying, and here comes a Buckeye fan to rub it in!" he must have thought.

When I finally said the words, "I am an ER doctor," my patient and his wife each gave me a look that defines the expression "a picture is worth a thousand words." I began to feel a sense of pride and, frankly, relief. It struck me that if I weren't an emergency physician, I would likely have been as scared as the patient. What if I were a psychiatrist, or even worse, a surgeon, with nary a scalpel to be found? After all, to most of the public a doctor is a doctor, and expectations and hopes aren't adjusted according to specialty. I was relieved by the fact that I was an emergency physician.

As it turned out, within a short time the gentleman was completely asymptomatic. The details of the case itself aren't particularly interesting to any of us practicing in our nation's emergency departments. Suffice it to say that he remained stable throughout the rest of the flight and did quite well.

We often dwell on the problems in our profession, which are numerous and complex. As problem solvers who demand much of ourselves, we concentrate on the negatives in an effort to change them for the better. We rarely stop to appreciate what's right with our profession. On that flight, however, I wasn't concerned about the malpractice crisis, decreasing reimbursement, EMTALA, drug seekers, honing my ultrasound skills, or my upcoming week of nights. I was focused solely on treating a very pleasant man who was in distress while providing comfort to his terrified wife, all while unknowingly serving as an example of our profession to the passengers watching.

Upon landing I shook his hand and wished him well while medics began placing him on monitors. His wife approached me, and then embraced me. She fought back tears as she clung tightly for several seconds and said, "Thank you so much." She really didn't need to say it: the hug said it all and more. A feeling of pride overwhelmed me, and to this day the memory of her embrace lifts my spirits, and if I really think about it, brings tears to my eyes.

When the call goes out, "I need a doctor!" whether on a plane, the side of a road, in a restaurant or theater, or every day in every city and town across the land in one of the nation's ER's, those best equipped to respond are emergency physicians. As a past and future patient, I extend my heartfelt gratitude to all of you, and as a colleague, let me say with utmost sincerity: I am proud to be one of you.

CHAPTER TWENTY-ONE

"I Think I'm Going to Die"

Chief complaint: Leg pain and shortness of breath

Bob was a 45-year-old man who arrived complaining of right leg pain and feeling slightly short of breath. He had been involved in an MVC (motor vehicle collision) a week before I saw him and had sustained a large cut on his left lower leg. He had also injured his back and had been admitted to a hospital in a neighboring state due to severe low back pain.

Bob was 6 feet tall but weighed close to five hundred pounds. His heart rate was 120, a bit fast but not surprising. His other vital signs were fine.

You may not have any idea where this is going, but any of my colleagues in emergency medicine who might read this already know what's wrong with Bob. He was a morbidly obese man who had recent trauma, was immobile due to back pain and hospitalization, complained of pain in the leg that wasn't injured, was short of breath, and was tachycardic.

Bob had a blood clot in his lung, or pulmonary embolus.

Pulmonary emboli are deadly. The most critical part of diagnosing them is suspecting them. In Bob's case, there was no doubt in my mind. I knew Bob had a PE, to the point that I immediately started treating him with an infusion of heparin, a blood thinner. I had no choice, actually, because Bob was too big for our scanners, so there was no way to get a diagnostic test to confirm my suspicion. I wasn't too concerned about that, as I felt quite confident that I knew exactly what was wrong with him.

During any patient encounter in the ER, my primary goal is to accurately diagnose and properly treat the patient. Customer service, patient satisfaction, the patient experience—whatever you want to call it—is icing on the cake, but what matters most is getting it right, correctly figuring out what's wrong and addressing it appropriately. I had done both quickly and efficiently.

Each time I checked on Bob, though, he continued to complain that he felt worse. We constantly monitored his vital signs, and there was never any significant change. Bob was clearly becoming more anxious, though.

Symptoms such as anxiety are landmines. They are also part of what distinguishes good clinicians from average or poor ones. A physician must maintain constant vigilance against minimizing these types of symptoms. These are classic problems you learn to handle during internship.

A nurse from the medical floor pages you in the middle of the night to tell you, "Mrs. MacDonald is really agitated tonight. Can I give her some Ativan or restrain her?" A less vigilant intern says "Sure, give her 2 mg of Ativan," and rolls over and goes back to sleep. A sharper one says, "Let me come see her first. I'll be right there."

Maybe Mrs. MacDonald is experiencing a drug reaction or side effect; maybe she's becoming psychotic from lack of normal sleep or being taken out of her familiar home environment; maybe she's hypoxic or brewing an infection; maybe something even worse. You'll never figure it out from your bed. You have to go look for yourself. One of my biggest pet peeves in medicine is when patients suffer from a doctor's laziness.

Knowing that full well, I also understood that Bob had a serious medical condition, so maybe it was normal for him to be anxious about it. His pulse oximetry remained normal; his heart rate was still fast but holding steady. He was breathing at about the same rate. I kept checking on him. He continued to look stable, but there was something about it I just didn't like.

Bob again complained that he felt more short of breath. Then he said it.

"I think I'm going to die."

That's when I thought to myself, "Fuck! Bob's going to die!"

"No, you're not." I told Bob. "Try to calm down. It's a good thing you came in when you did. We know what the problem is and we are treating you for it with the blood thinner. We're going to move you to a more comfortable bed soon." I said it as if I believed it, which is the way a patient wants and needs to hear it.

My internal voice was not convinced. I gave Bob a touch of Ativan to relax him a bit without affecting his respirations, even though I knew it wasn't really just anxiety causing him to feel this way.

I began to watch Bob even more closely, rarely stepping out of the room for more than a couple of minutes. I still had several other patients to tend to, but I was waiting for something to change, preferably for the better.

Ominously, Bob's breathing then became more labored. Bob spoke again.

"I'm going to die."

Those were Bob's last words. Within two minutes, he did.

Bob stopped breathing. All I could think at that moment was that I needed to intubate him to save him, but I knew that passing a tube in a man his size would not be easy. Fortunately, the difficult airway courses and CME

I'd completed paid off and the intubation went smoothly as CPR was performed. Revisiting this now, almost two decades later, I realize that the approach, diagnostic abilities and treatment options we utilize nowadays might possibly have saved Bob, yet people today still die from PE, so maybe not.

I continued to lead the resuscitation for a longer time than I probably should have, not wanting to give up, frustrated that I had known what was wrong with Bob the minute I saw him and had initiated the correct treatment right away, yet there I was coding him. I eventually acknowledged reality and pronounced Bob dead.

Just because you know exactly what the problem is and how to treat it doesn't mean patients don't die. Sometimes the patient knows that before we do. Bob told me he was going to die. I told him he wasn't. When the patient says they feel like they are going to die, always, always listen.

CHAPTER TWENTY-TWO

You're a Man, Right?

There are mommas' boys and then there are mommas' boys. Once a man reaches the age of legal adulthood, it should be considered socially acceptable to have your mommy bring you to the ER only under one of the following conditions:

1. You live alone, are unable to drive yourself to the ER, you don't own a phone, and you are too weak to crawl to the street to hitch a ride.
2. To identify your body.

If you're thirty-five and your mom came to the ER with you because you still live in her basement, where you spend most of your time managing a Fantasy Football league or searching Pornhub, and you let your mom answer most of my questions for you, someone needs to kick your ass.

If you were to ask my wife and daughter, they would tell you I'm one of the biggest feminists they know. I refuse to accept any less for my daughter than I would for my sons. Having said that, I do believe that women are the fairer sex, in every good way imaginable. I believe in chivalry. I believe in protecting women. I believe that while women have every right to serve in combat, I prefer that men kill each other in wars. After all, it is men who start them.

While we men consider ourselves tough, medicine has proven time and again that women are far tougher, and it's not even close. I'm not just talking about childbirth, though that's a solid example. I believe if men had the babies, the world would be a much smaller place, because you might fool some of us once, but none of us are falling for that a second time.

This was demonstrated to me in no uncertain terms at the births of my own children. I was 32 when my first child was born and was naïve enough to have considered myself a bit of a badass, if I did say so myself. I'd served in the Army, pulling many 24-hour shifts on guard duty and spending time in the field for days on little sleep. As noted previously, I took heavy course loads in college while working part-time. From the 3rd year of medical school through three years of residency, I had put in a tremendous number of work hours. Sleep was for wimps. I was one of those "I'll sleep when I'm dead" guys.

I had just started a night shift when my wife called to tell me it was time to go to the hospital. I got someone to cover the rest of my shift, then drove home and picked her up. We headed back to the hospital together, which was about a half-hour drive. I had to stop the car during each contraction because hitting a large pothole during labor was not particularly appreciated.

I started off strong as the attentive, doting and supportive father-in-waiting. Fast forward about eleven hours and my wife was still in labor as I slept on the other bed in her room. I was exhausted! She just kept going. Our son was born—I was awake for that, obviously—and the next morning the three of us were in the car again, this time with our brand-new baby in the car seat.

My wife was just warming up. As she waited for her milk to come in, recovered from the physical toll of childbirth, and watched over our newborn with the diligence of a soldier guarding the Tomb of the Unknown

Soldier, she didn't sleep for days. For days! I was bone-weary. I tried to keep up. "Come on, man. You got this," I'd tell myself. "But I'm so tired," I countered. The entire experience was a real eye-opener. It was the first time I learned about "nesting," an honest-to-goodness biological process that apparently gives women superpowers men can only dream about.

Women's toughness extends beyond birthing our young, however. Almost every patient I've ever seen faint while getting an immunization or witnessing something bloody or painful? A man. Don't believe me? Here are just a few examples of men behaving manly.

Chief complaint: Sunburn

A 19-year-old male arrived by ambulance. As I looked at his chief complaint as listed on the chart, "sunburn", I thought to myself, "Must be one hell of a sunburn to come in by ambulance."

I entered the room to find him sitting on the gurney in no apparent distress.

"Hi, I'm Dr. Duling, what brings you in today?"

"I have a sunburn."

"Does it hurt?"

"No. It was itching."

"Did you call the ambulance because it was itching?"

"Oh, no. The itching stopped after I took Benadryl."

"You lost me. If the itching had stopped, why did you call the ambulance?"

"I was afraid it would come back."

As I often do, I repeated a summary of the history back to him, just to make sure I had the story straight.

"You have a sunburn. It doesn't hurt. It was itching, which went away with Benadryl, but you were afraid the itching would come back, so you called 911 and came to the ER by ambulance?"

"Yes."

There is no other way to characterize this other than as a completely inappropriate waste of public resources. More to the point, though, this was supposedly a *man* we're talking about here. Calling an ambulance for phantom itching from a sunburn is about as pathetic as getting out of the draft because of phantom bone spurs.

Chief complaint: "I need a doctor's note."

A 19-year-old male presented to the ER who told me, "I have a cold." After examining him and confirming his suspicion, I explained that in fact nothing can be done for a cold other than over-the-counter cold remedies. He said, "Yes, I know." Then he told me that he needed a doctor's note, not for work or school, but for his friend's "kegger."

That's right—his friend was having a party, and the patient really didn't want to go, so he figured he'd pop into the ER and get a doctor's note stating he should not be drinking and partying with this cold. He was afraid that if he simply told his friend that he didn't want to go to the party, his friend would give him a hard time.

I asked him if he needed a work excuse; he told me he didn't have a job. He was on state assistance; taxpayers were funding his free trip to the ER to get a doctor's note to get out of the kegger.

Chief complaint: "I need some ibuprofen."

A 28-year-old male had just seen his dentist and was given prescriptions for Vicodin and penicillin for a tooth abscess. He was also instructed to use ibuprofen, however, and was now in the ER to get a prescription for ibuprofen.

"Ibuprofen is an over-the-counter medication. You can pick it up anywhere," I told him, somewhat surprised that any adult human being wouldn't know that.

"I know that," he retorted sarcastically. "I need a prescription so my Medicaid will pay for it."

Yes, a grown man came to the ER on the taxpayers' dime so that he wouldn't have to shell out the five bucks for a bottle of Advil. You would be shocked to know how often this happens. Lots of people would rather come to the ER and wait for three hours to get free ibuprofen rather than pay the $5 to pick some up from the store.

Chief complaint: "I think I overdosed."

A 17-year-old male presents by ambulance after being picked up from church camp. He had "overdosed."

"What did you take?" I asked, more by rote than actual concern, because I could tell from looking at him and his vital signs that he was completely fine.

"I drank three energy drinks and I felt really shaky," he informed me.

Considered in isolation, this comment may well have led me to think this kid needed to toughen up just a bit, but it was the other non-verbal communication going on in the room that truly told the story.

This 17-year-old boy, fresh from church camp, had a stuffed penguin with him. He referred to it as his "Pengi" and asked for a "blankie" for "Pengi." He then tucked the blanket up tight under the chin of his stuffed animal to keep it warm and safe.

You may be wondering, so I'll tell you. No, this kid didn't have special needs. It was rather obvious in talking to his parents that they had enabled this type of behavior.

I admit that the question going through my head lacked empathy and leaned toward judgmental. Should we pre-register this kid as a sex offender? It just felt like that's where things were headed.

Chief complaint: "I think I have an abscess"

A 52-year-old male complains of what he thinks is an abscess between his butt cheeks. He was lying on his side on the bed, already in a gown, and a woman accompanied him who was sitting in the chair at the far end of the room.

I asked, "How long have you had it?"

To answer the question, the woman leaped out of her seat and bolted toward us. She flipped his robe up, exposing his bare bottom, and *without gloves*, proceeded to spread his butt cheeks apart and show me the area in question. She pointed out how she had checked it a few times a day for the last four or five days and it didn't seem to be getting any better.

I could tell you the rest of the medical details at this point, but do they really matter? The only thing going through my head was how embarrassed I'd be if my wife had to do this for me.

I went back to my workstation and relayed the humor in this to my staff, to which one of them mentioned that she was "grossed out to think of his mom doing that."

"What?" I asked incredulously. "That's not his wife?"

"No," the tech told me. "It's his mom."

Just ew.

To be fair, there are men at the other end of the spectrum who are tough but not always too smart. I get it. I've been one of those men more than once. There's good reason why "Hold my beer" became a cliché. It's easy to look at the end result and *then* clearly see the potential for failure in any plan; hindsight is 20/20. As a guy, sometimes the vision of how the plan, if executed

132

flawlessly, just can't fail doesn't work out as we imagined. Thus another cliché: "It seemed like a good idea at the time."

Chief complaint: "I fell off my lawnmower"

A 43-year-old male complains of low back and left arm pain after falling off his lawnmower.

I figured he must have somehow fallen off his riding mower while doing his yard. Wrong.

Just when you thought motorsports couldn't get any more redneck than Nascar, along comes lawnmower racing, which at the time apparently commanded a fairly sizeable following. The "sport" was borne by men taking the blades off their riding mowers, adding more horsepower, and the next thing you knew you had two guys named Bubba in wife beaters with their beer guts resting against the seats of their lawnmowers as they drag raced for a six-pack of Bud Light and sheer pride.

If you can put wheels, skids or propellors on it, men will figure out a way to kill themselves with it. For many of us, it's not a Y chromosome, it's a "Y not?"

The patient told me, "These aren't stock mowers, Doc," in a tone he clearly thought would help me make sense of it all. "There's a big tuner market for lawnmowers. This thing *hauls ass*!"

I had a brief vision of a Hollywood blockbuster called "The Fast and the Fertilized".

This is one sport that will continue to be dominated by white guys, though I would pay to see a lawnmower with hydraulics and spinners.

CHAPTER TWENTY-THREE

Second Chances

<u>Chief complaint: "Not acting normally."</u>

Samuel was a 19-month-old boy who was brought in because his dad heard him fall out of his crib and he seemed "stunned" for a few minutes. Dad, clearly concerned and understandably anxious, said Samuel just sat there like he couldn't move, and wasn't making any sounds, "like he was just limp." He now seemed to be acting normally, according to Dad. He hadn't vomited and was able to eat and walk normally for his age.

On exam, Samuel was a cute little guy who seemed completely happy. He was sitting and smiling, playing with a block and taking a bottle. There was nothing abnormal about his exam or behavior. He seemed totally fine. I didn't really see the need for a big workup: kids who look this good generally don't have bad things going on.

After completing my evaluation, I sought Dad out.

"Hi, I'm Dr. Duling. You're Samuel's dad?"

"No, his mom is my girlfriend."

I reassured him that Samuel was fine and informed him that I didn't think we needed to do anything more. Since he was neither a parent nor legal guardian, though, I contacted Mom at work to tell her that Samuel looked great and that I didn't find anything to be concerned about. Mom sounded very nice on the phone. I asked if it was OK to discharge Samuel with her boyfriend. She told me her boyfriend was a great guy who watched the kids while she worked odd hours, and that she couldn't wait to get off work to see them both.

I discharged the boy with his mom's boyfriend. Samuel jumped up and ran out the door with him.

I picked up the next chart, finished an uneventful shift, and life went on.

Chief complaint: "Not responding."

I exited a patient room into the main corridor of our emergency department next to our resuscitation rooms just in time to see one of our nurses cradling a small child while running from the triage area. Few things in emergency medicine are more alarming than a nurse sprinting toward you with a motionless child in their arms. While hopefully imperceptible to everyone else there, I hesitated for just a second to clear every other thought from my head. This was the time for laser-sharp focus, not for hesitation or doubt. I took a deep breath and bolted toward the unresponsive child and the ultra-professional nurse, who acted as calm and cool as they come, though I could tell she was as concerned as I was.

Four-year-old children stop moving for one of two reasons: they have either exhausted every last bit of energy they can possibly squeeze out of their little bodies, or because something very, very bad is going on.

Tommy, the child in front of me, wasn't tired.

I immediately began assessing the situation. Tommy's eyes were open. That was a start. His chest moved slowly up and down as he breathed easily—also encouraging. In fact, as I listened to his chest and took note of his respirations, the nurse hooked him up to the pulse oximeter, which registered 99%.

His face was pale, but his skin was warm and dry, as it should be. His blood pressure was 88/60, pretty normal for his age, another reassuring fact. His heart was in a normal sinus rhythm with a rate in the 90's. Even his rectal temperature was normal. To look at his vital signs you'd think he was fine, but it was obvious that Tommy was anything but.

I searched for clues as to what would cause this change in his mental status. Had he sustained any sort of head trauma? There was no bruising or swelling on his head. Could he have ingested something: a pill he found on the floor or a dangerous cleanser or chemical found under the sink? Could his blood sugar be low? The nurse quickly checked it: 86, perfectly normal.

I continued to examine Tommy from head to toe. His neck was supple with no rigidity; no signs of meningitis, which could cause confusion and more profound changes in mental status. He had a normal exam of his chest, abdomen, pelvis, and extremities.

Tommy's only abnormalities were neurologic. He just laid there, limp and floppy. While we poked his arms to draw blood and start an IV, he didn't even flinch, which is never normal for a four-year-old. He had normal reflexes, though, and his toes bent downward when scraping the soles of his feet, another normal reflex. He wasn't paralyzed; it was as if he had no desire to move whatsoever. His pupils were equal, round, and reactive to light.

I tried to look at his fundi, the back of the inside of his eyes. His pupils were fairly small, though, and it was tough to see a good portion of the retinae. I didn't see anything grossly abnormal.

I again went over his differential diagnosis, the list of possible causes. "OK, now think!" I urged myself. By this time things were a little calmer, both in the resuscitation room and inside my brain, as it seemed that Tommy wasn't dying, at least on the spot. Something was seriously wrong, though. What was it? He didn't look septic; his heart rate, blood pressure, and temperature were completely normal.

He didn't exhibit signs of any specific toxidrome I could think of. A toxidrome is a collection of symptoms and signs commonly associated with a certain type of poison or toxin. For example, organophosphates are used as pesticides on farms, and on a rare occasion you might see a farmer come in with some combination of the following findings: severe headache, runny eyes and nose, confusion, muscle twitching, vomiting, diarrhea, incontinence, pinpoint pupils, a slow heart rate, and possibly more severe symptoms including paralysis and the inability to breathe. That's the toxidrome for organophosphate, or nerve agent, poisoning.

Other specific toxidromes are identifiable for drugs like stimulants such as cocaine or amphetamines or for other substances like tricyclic antidepressants, heroin, anticholinergics, etc.

Tommy didn't exhibit signs of any specific toxidrome, nor of sepsis or meningitis. It was time to run some blood work and get a CT scan of his head. It had been less than ten minutes since Tommy was carried back to the resuscitation room because it was thought he may be dying. It's amazing how ten minutes can change someone's life. Sometimes it doesn't even take that long.

As I ordered the tests, I sought out the parents to bring them up to speed. The child was accompanied by a man who looked instantly familiar. I'm not one of those people who never forgets a face, but something about this guy's face was familiar, though I couldn't place it. I explained to him what we were doing for Tommy and asked how he was related.

"I'm his mom's boyfriend."

Something clicked inside me. The little voice began questioning; where had we heard that before?

"Tell me a little about what you've noticed or seen with Tommy today," I prompted him.

"I don't know. He kind of tripped and fell, and then it was like he just went limp."

Total bullshit. No way he came in unresponsive because he tripped and fell.

My little voice started piecing it together. "Have you ever heard a story like that before?" the voice asked me. I had, in fact, just a couple of months prior. What was it?

Wait a minute! I had seen a younger child who had fallen out of his crib and had presented with a history of altered mental status, though that child seemed fine when I saw him. I distinctly recalled the man who had brought the child in describing him as "just going limp" as well. Come to think of it, that guy wasn't the child's father, either. The voice was feeding me information as quickly as I could process it now.

The man who brought that child in two months ago was also mom's boyfriend, and mom had been at work at that time, too. That man was... the same man standing before me.

The wave of emotions that came over me at that moment was crushing. This man had brought two children in to see me in a two-month span. The first child had been fine, but now Tommy lay in my resuscitation room as a victim of what I strongly suspected was child abuse.

I knew the statistics. Boyfriends who are not the child's father are far more likely to abuse them. ER doctors are always on the lookout for child abuse.

I was able to recognize child abuse in Tommy's case because of the severity of his presentation and his mom's boyfriend's bullshit explanation for it, but when I had seen Samuel two months prior, I had not identified any red flags.

I transferred Tommy to a local Children's Hospital, and when giving report to the accepting ER doc there, I detailed my concerns regarding abuse. I didn't say anything to the boyfriend but did relay my concerns to Tommy's and Samuel's mother by phone. I couldn't imagine the feelings one experiences when leaving your children with someone you absolutely trust only to find out that your trust has been betrayed in the most horrific way possible.

Confirming my fears, Tommy's head CT showed small hemorrhages in the occipital and frontal lobes. The findings added up to shaken baby syndrome. When a child is violently shaken back and forth, it causes the brain to be smashed against the front of the skull, then the back, in a series of blows that induce bleeding and lead to disruption of normal brain activity. That explained why there was nothing else abnormal on Tommy's examination. His brain was essentially stunned. I was thrilled to see that before leaving our emergency department Tommy began to move around and even talk. The damage was transient, and he would go on to recover fully.

The boyfriend later confessed and was convicted of child abuse, though I never heard what his punishment was. Mine was knowing I'd missed an opportunity to spot a child abuser two months prior, though I was glad I helped nail the bastard when given a second chance.

I can't help but wonder whether I've failed to spot child abuse on other occasions. Sometimes my little voice talks to me while I am evaluating a child or interviewing the parents. "Look at that guy," I'll think. "He's looked pissed off the whole time he's been here. He looks pissed off at his kid...his wife...me. How much you want to bet he beats his wife and kids?" I can almost visualize the man's hand raised to strike his child or wife, but unless I see something concrete, or a patient wants to tell me something, there's nothing I can do.

I once got a vibe from a patient's boyfriend that he seemed like an abusive dick, so I invented a reason for him to leave the room so I could ask her about it. She adamantly denied that he abused her. After her broken arm was splinted, I discharged her. A few minutes later, one of our techs came back from lunch and said, "You know that woman who was in room 5? I just saw her boyfriend beating the crap out of her in their car. I'm calling the police." Police responded and hauled his ass off to jail.

What makes identifying child abuse even more difficult is that when someone brings a child to the ER because of "suspected abuse," sometimes it's just a ploy in a bitter divorce or custody dispute. Mom or Dad will bring the kid in on Sunday night after a weekend with the other parent.

"I want it documented that he was abused," they'll say, as if getting this into the medical record somehow makes it legal fact.

Another form of child abuse is using your children to support your habits. I once saw a 13-year-old girl who had injured her foot a week prior to her visit to my ER. It was still slightly bruised but not swollen. The girl did not appear to be in any distress whatsoever and was walking on the foot just fine. Her mom asked if she could have anything for pain. I told her that the girl should use Tylenol or ibuprofen. Mom said she was using both but that the child was still crying in pain at night. Mom said, "She had Vicodin before and it seemed to work real good."

I told Mom there was no way I would prescribe Vicodin for a week-old sprain. When our nurse tried to discharge the patient she quickly returned because mom asked for some T3's (Tylenol with codeine) for the girl. In a moment of weakness, in part because I was tired of arguing with them and just wanted them to leave, in part because patient satisfaction scores have become surrogates for distinguishing "good doctors" from "bad doctors," and in part because I had several other patients to see, I gave the girl a prescription for eight T3's.

About an hour later, the pharmacy called to tell me that the mother had filled prescriptions for over 500 Percocet tablets that month alone. I told the pharmacy to cancel my prescription. Codeine has since been proven ineffective and problematic, so most of us haven't prescribed it in many years.

Another mother tried to get me to prescribe six months' worth of Ritalin for each of her two children who "both had ADHD." As her children sat beside her, very well-behaved for their ages, I wondered if she really thought that I didn't know that Ritalin was used in the production of methamphetamines.

We've all heard and/or expressed the sentiment that you need a license to drive a car but not to be a parent. Based on what I've seen, a lot of people shouldn't be allowed to do either.

CHAPTER TWENTY-FOUR

Stress

"The first thing we do, let's kill all the lawyers."
Shakespeare, from King Henry VI

You may be familiar with this definition of stress: the confusion created when one's mind overrides the body's basic desire to choke the living shit out of some asshole who desperately deserves it.

Chief complaint: "I got dizzy and felt like I was going to pass out."

During the middle of a fairly routine and uneventful shift, I was summoned by my charge nurse, Kylie, to witness a patient signing out against medical advice. The patient was a 79-year-old male attorney who had arrived by ambulance after experiencing near-syncope ("almost" passing out) at his law office. He was accompanied by his two sons who were both attorneys as well. His older son's first priority upon having his father arrive at an emergency room by ambulance was to make sure that no one from the ER treated his father. He insisted on speaking with "whoever is in charge" and proceeded to inform the charge nurse that no ER physician was to treat his father. He insisted that his father's personal physician, Dr. Jack Mickelson, be summoned immediately to evaluate him.

Our charge nurse tried to explain that things just didn't work that way in an ER. Still, every patient has the right to refuse treatment if competent. Given the fact that the patient and his sons were all lawyers, and given the initially adversarial and hostile tone of the encounter, the charge nurse wanted to ensure that a physician was involved in the process right away.

You can imagine what went through my mind as Kylie explained the situation to me. It was no personal offense to me; I hadn't even laid eyes on the man yet. The insinuation in such a request, though, was clearly that as far as this patient and his family were concerned, an ER physician was not competent enough to treat him. Who knew what the source of the sentiment could be? For all intents and purposes, it didn't matter.

When someone arrives in the ER and starts demanding VIP treatment while the place is packed with plenty of other patients who require urgent attention, and the first thing out of their mouths is an insult, you can imagine how excited the entire staff is about the notion of providing personalized and exceptional service.

The most important part of signing someone out against medical advice is not merely having them sign an AMA form. It is providing an informed refusal of treatment. The patient needed to understand exactly what might happen to him if he refused testing or treatment. I decided to go the extra yard in this case and tried to determine exactly what the problem was. I went to his bedside and introduced myself.

"Hello, sir. I'm Dr. Duling. I'm one of the ER doctors here. I understand you almost passed out?"

His son immediately interjected. "Look, this is nothing against you guys. We want him to be seen by his cardiologist who is familiar with his care."

"Who is his cardiologist?" I inquired.

"Dr. Mickelson," his son said as if annoyed that I wouldn't somehow know that already.

"I don't know him," I replied. "Where does he practice?"

"At this hospital," his son said more sharply, again as if this was exactly why he didn't want some dumb ER doctor taking care of his dad.

"I've been here several years, and I've never heard that name. I can look him up," I responded.

"Well, he was on staff here the last time he saw Dad."

"How long ago was that?"

"Maybe seven years ago."

"Let's get to what brought you in," I offered, in an attempt to get the visit on track. I explained, "Private physicians virtually never come to the ER to see their patients. They can't just close their office practice down every time one of their patients comes to the ER, as you can imagine."

"Of course," his older son acknowledged.

"Why don't you let me get things started, and I will call your doctor right away to make sure that the testing we do is OK by him. How does that sound?"

Having to suck up to such a pompous ass as this guy, and particularly his sons, made my blood start to boil.

"Okay, that sounds fine," his son conceded. The patient agreed.

After interviewing and examining the patient, I told him my concerns.

"Because of the dizziness you experienced and the fact that you almost passed out, I think we need to do a CT scan of your brain, as well as an ECG and some blood work."

I looked up his cardiologist, who had retired a few years earlier, so I called our cardiologist on call and explained the situation, to which he replied, "Hey man, you're the one seeing him. Do what you need to do."

I translated this to the patient as, "Sir, unfortunately Dr. Mickelson has retired, but I did speak with one of our cardiologists, a very smart guy—you'd like him—who thought that our initial plan sounded good. Should we go ahead with it?"

The patient agreed and was eventually taken for a CT scan of his brain. The CT report read as follows:

Atrophy.
Old lacunar infarct.
Brain otherwise normal.

Translation:

The brain shrinks with age (atrophy), a fairly common finding in the elderly.

At some point the patient had a small stroke (the old lacunar infarct), meaning that a small portion of the brain was dead. The patient never even knew he had it.

The brain otherwise looked normal.

Here's what I told the patient and his sons:

"Sir, your CT scan shows a couple of things we often see with age, but otherwise looks OK. I am very concerned about your symptoms, though, and I think we should keep you in the hospital overnight and have our neurologist take a look at you."

Here's what I *wanted* to say:

"Sir, your CT scan shows that your brain is unusually small, that you are partially brain-dead, and given your symptoms, it appears that the rest of your brain isn't working very well either. The good news is that you should continue to do well as an attorney."

That is stress.

CHAPTER TWENTY-FIVE

Performing at a Time of Crisis

As a young boy growing up in the 1970s, aside from family and playing with my friends, I loved three things above all others: Ohio State football, Led Zeppelin, and cars/motorcycles. A 16th birthday was intended for only one purpose: to head down to the DMV and get your driver's license.

Back in the day, before airbags existed and when no one called CPS for letting a kid sit in the front seat, I'd watch my dad intently as he drove our car, which was a stick. I'd go through the motions of rowing through the gears in my head. My mental practice paid off when we went on our annual camping trip during the summer I was twelve.

Mr. Baker was one of my dad's best friends from high school. He owned an old Jeep he would tow behind his motorhome up to the Canoe Camps along the Muskegon River near Harrison, Michigan. We spent one glorious week each summer riding dirt bikes, canoeing, bathing in the river, sleeping in tents or campers, and laughing endlessly beside a bonfire each night.

One evening, Mr. Baker piled three other boys and me into the Jeep for some off-roading on the primitive roads and dirt trails. He let his son, just a few months older than me, drive for a bit, then he asked me if I wanted to try it.

"Yes, I do!" I shouted.

As far as anyone knew, I hadn't ever driven a car. I failed to disclose that, on occasion, when my parents were at work, I'd been known to slowly back our Jeep Cherokee out of the driveway and take it for a quick spin around the block. The Cherokee had a manual transmission, which gave me just enough experience to feel rather confident I could drive the Jeep at least as well as his son, Robbie, had.

After settling in behind the wheel, Mr. Baker warned me, "Be careful. Sometimes when you turn hard to the left the steering wheel locks."

"OK," I said while thinking, "Whatever that means."

I expertly shifted into first gear and slowly released the clutch until the Jeep was propelled smoothly forward. Over the next few minutes, I shifted several times, keeping the RPM right where they needed to be, and was unquestionably impressing Mr. Baker and the other boys, who felt so comfortable with my smooth-shifting and reasonable ability to avoid potholes on the dirt roads that they'd decided to stand up in the back seat and hold onto the roll bar.

As we approached an offshoot of the "main" road, Mr. Baker said, "Take a left here."

I slowed and downshifted, cranking the steering wheel hard to the left. As I tried to straighten the wheels, the steering wheel wouldn't turn. Mr. Baker reiterated, "The steering wheel is locked. Stop the car."

Instead, I panicked. Frustrated that the wheel wouldn't turn in the direction I wanted, I actually sped up as we continued making a hard left, now blazing through heavier brush, accelerating until I hit a tree. The boys in the back lurched forward against the roll bar.

Fortunately, no one was injured, but the damage to Mr. Baker's Jeep was plainly evident: a semilunar concavity in the middle of the front bumper. Deciding that having a Jeep that couldn't turn left might not be the best vehicle to let the boys drive, Mr. Baker decided that was enough driving the Jeep for the rest of the trip.

To this day, the story is good for some hearty laughs on my account, which is understandable and expected. What no one knows, though, is that moment was the first time I thought about why people fold under pressure, particularly why *I* had choked.

I was upset with myself that, even at the age of twelve, I wasn't composed enough to listen and follow simple instructions that would have avoided the entire problem. Instead, I froze. I wasn't able to hear, process information, or think. I didn't act because I panicked.

A few years later, after witnessing the strength my father showed by identifying my cousin's body and protecting his sister and brother-in-law from that horrific imagery, I was more acutely aware of his ability to manage a crisis than I would have been without this insight gained by crashing Mr. Baker's Jeep.

During my time in the military, I became interested in what made leaders great, or at least effective. I read the principles laid out in FM 22-100, the Army's field manual on military leadership. Of all the leadership philosophies and traits, without question the most effective is to lead by example. The leadership principle that imparts the ability to plan and execute at the highest level, however, is to teach everyone on your team to lead.

Given my early curiosity about decision-making and crisis management, my exploration of the foundation of good leadership, and their obvious relevance to my chosen profession of emergency medicine, over the course of my career I've studied and given a lot of thought to these aspects of being an ER doctor. Most doctors are in the position of being team leaders, yet we don't often teach leadership skills to doctors.

I don't believe in "born leaders," as the notion implies that you don't need to learn anything to be a leader, when nothing could be further from the truth. Leadership, performance under pressure, and management of a crisis are learned skills.

I don't claim to be an expert on leadership. My own skills and shortcomings as a leader are best assessed by those I have had the privilege of leading, not by me. I do know that I make the effort to employ lessons I've learned from the many effective leaders I've known in my life, but every serviceable leader is potentially one bad decision away from becoming a terrible leader.

In my experience, the steps to surviving, managing, and leading or even thriving in a crisis are: Prepare, Manage, Accept.

Prepare

I don't know who said it first, but we've all probably heard of the 7 P's: Proper prior planning prevents piss-poor performance. Like Murphy's Law, it's a universal truth.

The people we look to in a moment of crisis spend a great deal of time preparing to implement their crisis management plans.

Take firefighters. I've met many firefighters over the years. I don't deny that most firefighters have an intrinsic personality disorder that compels them to run toward danger rather than away from it. A group of kids riding their bikes come upon a house fire. Most of the kids want to watch. The future firefighter says, "Come on, let's get closer and see if anyone needs help."

A firefighter might be predisposed to want to help out of a sense of empathy or caring, but they don't know the first damn thing about how to put out a fire until they *prepare* to do the job. Fire training academies help prepare them to manage the crisis of entering a burning building to save life and property.

How hot are fires? Does it matter what's burning? Other than smoke and flame, are there any hazards specific to different types of fires? How can you tell if a structure is about to collapse? What are the techniques of fighting fires? Of extricating victims?

Firefighters train extensively to learn the principles of their craft, then work alongside veterans who impart real-world wisdom to continue their preparation.

As an exercise, think about someone or a group of people who impress you with the way they are able to make something difficult look easy. The only way that happens is by putting in the time and effort to prepare.

Manage

Management of a crisis encompasses three distinct elements that can occur separately, simultaneously, or overlap.

Don't Panic
Think
Act

Not panicking doesn't always equate to remaining calm. One might be excited, anxious or afraid. *Don't panic* means not being so overwhelmed in the moment that you can't think clearly. Focusing our mental energy and problem-solving ability—*thinking*—offers our best chance of success. If we can avoid panicking and think clearly, we need only to execute the plan we've come up with—to *act*.

As one of the more dramatic and vivid examples of managing a crisis, I enter into evidence Exhibit A: the Miracle on the Hudson. On January 15, 2009, US Airways Flight 1549 had just taken off from LaGuardia Airport in New York City headed to North Carolina. The aircraft hit a flock of birds while climbing, causing a loss of all power, turning the Airbus A320 into a glider. 155 souls were on board.

The plane was skillfully piloted to a water landing in the Hudson River. Everyone on board survived.

It was no miracle. It must be recognized that the biggest factor in the unbelievably ecstatic ending in the river that day was the first step in this paradigm—preparation.

Captain Chesley "Sully" Sullenberger had logged nearly 20,000 flight hours, had been a fighter pilot, and was also a glider pilot and an aviation safety expert. First Officer Jeff Skiles was likewise an experienced pilot. Their vast experience, knowledge, and training prepared them for that moment. Without preparation, January 15th might mark a tragic anniversary for 155 families.

In terms of managing the crisis—not panicking, thinking, acting—the pilots ran through their options, chose the only one they deemed feasible, and acted immediately to execute their plan.

As an ER doctor, I must take a moment to editorialize about the way Sully did not panic, which is a tremendous understatement.

When a critically ill patient comes to *my* workplace, ER doctors, nurses and staff do our very best not to panic—to remain calm yet decisive as our team manages a resuscitation or whatever challenge is on the gurney in front of us. As we do so, our lives are usually not on the line, though Covid-19 has changed this dynamic. We're pretty good at not panicking, thinking, and acting. The people I work with are amazing under pressure.

But come on! Really, Sully? *You* are potentially going down with the plane, yet you remain *that* calm, cool and collected? Give the rest of us a break, man!

You heard it on the radio communication when Capt. Sullenberger said, "We're gonna be in the Hudson." But it was the *way* he said it.

I confess that this next part is completely fabricated, but this is the dialogue I imagined going through Sully's head during Flight 1549:

"Wheels up. What a nice day. Hmmm hmmm hmm hmm hmm," he hums to himself as the plane climbs and the landing gear retracts. "Look, some birdies. That's nice. Ooh, looks like we clipped a few of you. Hope you're OK there, little fellas. Ha—look at that—engine lights are on. Better get the oil changed when I get back. Can't be too cautious. Boy, it sure is nice up here when it's quiet like this. Really lets you clear your head and think."

Around this time, he mentions to an air traffic controller, "We're gonna be in the Hudson." I then picture him telling the passengers in the cabin, "Hi there folks, this is Sully, your Captain speaking. We're currently cruising at an altitude of 800, 700… let's call it 600 feet. If you look out both sides of the aircraft, you're going to have a spectacular view of the Hudson. We're going to go ahead and postpone our beverage service. Oh, and, uh, just for kicks, let's pretend we're all on the Oprah show. If you look under your seats, I've given you all a flotation device! Everyone grab one and show it to your seatmates, then just hold on to it real tight."

From an ER doc, mad, mad, mad respect, Captain Sully.

Accept

The most neglected portion of crisis management is accepting the consequences. We need to understand that despite our best effort to prepare, not panic, think and act, things still may not turn out as we planned or hoped. In fact, things might end disastrously. It's possible that a misstep on our part plays a role in a suboptimal outcome.

Teddy Roosevelt once said, "In any moment of decision the best thing you can do is the right thing; the next best thing you can do is the wrong thing; the worst thing you can do is nothing."

Hard choices have to be made in life. There's no way around it. Consider the math. You are confronted with an agonizing, potentially life-altering decision. It could go either way—there's a 50/50 chance that your choice will work out as you intend.

This gives you a 1 in 2 chance of making the correct decision, right? Now, let's say you are confronted with a second, similar choice with the same odds. Then a third. In the course of your lifetime, do you think you've made three tough decisions? If you have, the odds that you've made all three of them correctly are 1 in 8. It's simple probability.

If you flip a coin three times, the odds of getting three heads are calculated this way:

$$\frac{1}{2} \times \frac{1}{2} \times \frac{1}{2} = 1/8$$

That means there's an 87.5% chance that you'll get at least one tail, or—extrapolating these odds to decision-making—that one of your three decisions will be wrong. Think about this mathematical fact and how it applies to your life and everyone around you.

Firefighters flocked up the stairs in the Twin Towers on 9/11 because they were well-prepared, they didn't panic, they thought about what they should do, and they acted with everything they had. No one anticipated that the heat would destroy the structural integrity of the building. Their attempt at crisis management ended disastrously and tragically. In my opinion, none of them were natural born leaders or natural crisis managers—they *earned* that distinction through their preparation and their management. They were undeniably, naturally heroic—on that point there is no debate. We understand why their efforts failed, and we deeply admire why they acted as they did. They died giving everything they had in an effort to save the lives of people they didn't know—what an amazing legacy.

We should attempt to consider the decisions of others in the same light, and to extend to family, friends, or complete strangers that which is sorely lacking in today's society: grace.

Hindsight is 20/20. It's easy to know what the correct choice was after you know the results. We should judge the actions of others based on whether it was reasonable to choose as they did with the information in hand at the time the decision was made.

More wisdom from Teddy Roosevelt contends with this issue directly.

"It is not the critic who counts; not the man who points out how the strong man stumbles, or where the doer of deeds might have done them better. The credit belongs to the man who is actually in the arena, whose face is marred by dust and sweat and blood; who strives valiantly; who errs and comes short again and again, because there is no effort without error and shortcoming; but who does actually strive to do the deeds; who knows great enthusiasms, the great devotions; who spends himself in a worthy cause; who at the best knows in the end the triumph of high achievement, and who, at the worst, if he fails, at least fails while daring greatly, so that his place shall never be with those cold and timid souls who know neither victory nor defeat."

I have had the privilege of working side by side with many women and men in the arena. They've earned my utmost respect not because they're always right, rather because they strive valiantly and dare greatly. Nothing more should be asked of any of us.

Caveats to Performing in a Crisis

The ability to manage one type of crisis doesn't translate to proficiency in managing a different form of crisis.

I'm an ER doc. I don't know the first thing about fighting fires. You either have special expertise on a subject matter or you don't. It may be true that your skill set enables you to coordinate a team and deploy the expertise of others in the most efficacious manner, but in order to perform each task in a crisis, one needs to prepare for that task.

A good example of this is a Special Operations team, in which several members of the team are well-versed and extremely prepared in weapons, demolitions, small unit tactics, tactical first aid and other skills. If one member of the team goes down, another can fill his/her place. This level of teamwork and performance doesn't happen by hiring a bunch of born leaders and having someone wing it when one of them goes down; it is the result of training and preparing every member of the team to be proficient in each of the tasks.

A corollary is that if you want to be a person who performs well in more than one type of crisis situation, you need to prepare for each and develop a plan and any skills you need that will enable you to not panic, think and act when the time comes.

Crises come in all shapes and sizes.

Your house is on fire. Your mother was just diagnosed with Alzheimer's. A tree fell on your house during a storm. You lost your job. There's an active shooter in your workplace. You have cancer and just learned you have six months to live.

Crises can unquestionably bring with them pain, suffering, tragedy, and profound sadness. They are also opportunities, many of which can be foreseen and planned for, because we should expect that life will throw us a few curves along the way, and we are operating under the advantage of knowing the endpoint for all of us. Acknowledging it and preparing for it ourselves, rather than leaving it to our families and loved ones to figure out on their own, are acts of love.

As an example, I know that my unexpected death would present a crisis for my family. I've prepared for this by maintaining a document detailing what steps my wife and children could take to make the painful transition to their next chapter of life just a bit easier. I've updated it every couple of years, most recently when Covid-19 hit. I know the grief would be overwhelming. I want to limit the chaos of my family having to sort everything out on their own by taking a few simple steps to prepare in advance.

As such, I gathered key documents into one place, I detailed our accounts, assets, names and numbers of people to contact, left clear wishes as to what to do with my remains, and discussed all of this with my family. In the first weeks of Covid-19, I went so far as to purchase an urn. I don't care if my wife were to buy a different one, but it serves as an example of one little thing she doesn't need to think about when she's hurting most.

Grace

I reiterate this point because its importance cannot be overstated. If you ask me, this is perhaps our greatest current failing as human beings—our inability to extend grace both to those we love and to strangers. We tend to demonize anyone who doesn't share our world view or who might dare to try to solve a problem in a manner different than we would choose.

We crucify a politician for a stance he or she held twenty years ago which is currently unpopular. We point out an error in judgement or execution as if ever getting anything wrong should disqualify us from being involved in future discussions and problem-solving efforts. It is a ridiculous standard that none of us can meet.

Sometimes mistakes are made that can't be corrected, with permanent, devastating results. When that occurs, our punishment as human beings is having to live with the "what ifs," wondering why things couldn't have gone differently. Our character is revealed, however, by what we choose to do with that insight. Do we use it to prepare so we are not caught off guard in a similar situation in the future? Or do we let it destroy our lives and those around us? We need to learn to cut ourselves some slack and extend a generosity of spirit to those around us.

Think of what kind of place the world could be if we learned to appreciate the best efforts of others, made with the best intentions in mind, even if the results fell short of our expectations.

As Sam Cooke sang, what a wonderful world this would be.

CHAPTER TWENTY-SIX

A Buckeye Named Maury

In the middle of a typically busy ER shift, I signed up to see the next patient. When I entered the exam room, I found an older man sitting in a wheelchair and immediately noticed his hat: a gray hat with red and white lettering that read, "Ohio State Buckeyes 2002 National Champions". I asked him, "Are you a Buckeye, sir?" He responded proudly, "You bet I am."

Maury and I were in Washington State, some 2,415 miles and an estimated 36 hours by car from Columbus, Ohio, according to MapQuest. Maury was 78 years old, 34 years older than I was, which also happened to be the number of years between Ohio State's two consensus national championships in 1968 and 2002. Buckeye fans tend to remember such facts.

We immediately began to talk Ohio State football, as any two Buckeyes who still had a pulse would. I listened in amazement as Maury told me he had attended The Ohio State University from 1950–1954: back when it was known simply as OSU. As the dates registered in my mind, I had to ask.

"Maury, that would mean you were a student at Ohio State during the Snow Bowl..."

I didn't even get the question out before he told me, "I was there."

I was officially in awe. As far as I was concerned, Maury was a rock star. His mind was razor sharp and filled with facts and details.

"It was the 25th of November 1950. You know, Thanksgiving is on the 25th this year." He proceeded to tell me about barely being able to see Vic Janowicz's field goal that gave Ohio State its first and only points. You could hear the melancholy in his voice when he said, "I decided to leave my seat and get to the restroom right before the half. I heard the crowd groaning and discovered that I had missed Michigan blocking our punt for a touchdown, the only one of the game." Michigan won the Snow Bowl, and six decades later Maury was still sore about it. Now *that's* a Buckeye.

During Maury's sophomore year, Ohio State got a new football coach. His name was Wayne Woodrow "Woody" Hayes.

Maury graduated from Ohio State in 1954 with a degree in foreign languages, having studied Russian, French and German while enrolled in ROTC. He became an officer in the Infantry and began a long career in the U.S. Army, serving in Germany and Korea as well as a stint in Vietnam.

What was Maury's favorite war story? He was in Vietnam in 1968 when Woody Hayes was visiting the troops there. Maury met and shook hands with Coach Hayes and asked him how good the Bucks were going to be that year. Woody told him, "If we can get by Purdue, we might be pretty good." He asked Coach Hayes who the quarterback was going to be. "A young man named Rex Kern," Woody informed him. As it turned out, the Buckeyes beat Purdue 13–0 that season and Woody was right: the 1968 team was pretty good, beating a running back named O.J. Simpson and USC in the Rose Bowl to win the national championship.

Maury had the good fortune to see Woody again in 1969, this time in Columbus. Woody Hayes deeply admired and respected those who fought and died to defend this country, and Maury was military through and through. The night we met in the emergency room, he was wearing fatigues, having survived both a career in the Army and the Ten Year War between Woody Hayes and Bo Schembechler.

Military service was a cornerstone of Maury's family. Maury's father, Maurice Sr., was a career Army officer who served in the Pacific in World War II. His brother Bill was a student at Ohio State for a quarter before attending the Naval Academy and serving a career as a Naval officer, commanding four warships and a large destroyer squadron. His other brother Fritz (OSU Class of '57) served in the Army before embarking on a career in television and radio in Columbus, achieving notoriety as "Fritz the Nite Owl" while hosting Nite Owl Theater on WBNS-TV from 1974–1991.

I was taken aback at the connection I instantly felt with Maury. He was an engaging man with a magnetic personality who could have told stories all night. Our encounter seemed richer and more meaningful than such a brief patient encounter typically would. While I have been a Buckeye all my life, my short time with Maury demonstrated to me just how strong the bond among all Buckeyes is.

Maury was also a tough old guy, so he very matter-of-factly told me that he was dying. Maury had cancer and was in hospice. As we talked about the upcoming Miami game, he acknowledged that this football season would be his last. He said, "It's kind of a tough deal, but I'm man enough to take it."

Our visit lasted all too briefly, and Maury went home.

As his caregiver wheeled him out of the emergency room, Maury said goodbye the only way that seemed appropriate, by pumping his fist into the air and shouting:

"GO BUCKS!"

A couple of weeks later, I was thinking about Maury and decided to pay him a visit. We spent a couple of hours talking about everything from his long military career to my short one to, of course, the Buckeyes. I asked Maury if he'd mind if I brought my sons to watch the Penn State game with him, as my daughter was still a bit young. We were both excited about the idea but had to wait a few weeks. When I called a few days before the game to firm up plans, I learned that Maury had died as only a hardcore Buckeye like him would: on a bye week.

I know he would have loved to see Ohio State earn their seventh pair of gold pants in a row a few weeks later.

I had the opportunity to meet his brothers, who were with him at the end. They were warm and gracious, and they gave me a few things of Maury's to give to my kids that they still treasure. From time to time when some minor adversity would come up my then-teenage son would say, "It's OK, I'm man enough to take it."

It is the greatest privilege of medicine to share some of life's moments with patients and their families. Some of those moments are difficult, which make the time we have with each other as human beings more precious and meaningful.

CHAPTER TWENTY-SEVEN

Distributive Justice

I can't write a book about emergency medicine without touching on the topic of health care as a right. As a society, we desperately need to have a critically important debate about health care, but these days it seems we can no longer engage in civil discourse with people with whom we disagree, so we don't even bother trying to solve difficult problems in this country anymore.

Perhaps some members of Congress should function more like ER doctors. I promise you we could do a better job. Check out the administration of most hospitals these days and you'll often find an ER doctor in there somewhere. Why? Because we do the simple things really well. We work and play well with others. We do more with less. Not solving the problem isn't an option for us, so we usually figure out a fairly decent solution. It may not be perfect, but we'll bust our asses to come up with something workable.

While earning my degree in philosophy with particular interest in medical ethics, I wrote my Honors Thesis about the concept of national health insurance. I'm actually not a fan of Medicare for all, but I do believe that health care is a right of every citizen. The Declaration of Independence promised us life, liberty, and the pursuit of happiness. These were deemed to be unalienable rights. How can one be promised life if we aren't going to care for someone who is ill? How is continuing to allow Americans to go bankrupt because they got sick not morally reprehensible?

I can't enjoy life or liberty or pursue happiness if I need emergency surgery and it costs me six months' pay. And if that is six months of my pay as a physician, it is years' worth of pay for many people. This is a ridiculous burden for anyone in one of the wealthiest countries in human history.

I am in my fifties, having made a good living for over twenty years. I've stashed some money in my 401k and have some equity in my home. By a strict accounting analysis, I'd be considered better off than most, but it sure doesn't feel like it, and all it would take to destroy my family's financial well-being is for me to get cancer or any other long-term debilitating disease. Just like that, a career, a home, my kids' college funds, our financial security in our golden years—every bit of financial "security" we've achieved—would be spent in a matter of months to maybe a few years. It is easily imaginable that by the time I turn 60 years of age I could be destitute and end up homeless, leaving my family with nothing.

I don't tell this cautionary tale to invoke pity for the "rich doctor." I am merely pointing out that if I am at risk of financial devastation due to illness or injury, so is over 90% of the population. I am pissed about it, because after two decades as a doctor, I don't think I should have to lose sleep over this fact. I can only imagine how terrified a young family with less means than my own must be in this day and age. It is obscene. It is wrong.

To fix it, we'd need to have some difficult conversations which would require a level of maturity and rationality that our country lacks. We need to talk about whether we should be spending an enormous amount of our finite health care resources caring for elderly patients at the end of life while we allow millions of citizens to go without health care altogether. We must achieve a deeper understanding of what we should or should not pay for and why.

Health care should be strongly rooted in utilitarianism, a philosophy based on the belief that we should use public resources to do the greatest good for the greatest number of people. As Spock said, "the needs of the many outweigh the needs of the few."

Health care is an example of the concept of distributive justice. We should think of health care as having a certain amount of goods. How can we most fairly distribute these goods to everyone? Some will undoubtedly need more than others. If we don't happen to need much, we should consider ourselves quite fortunate for our good health. As we were taught in kindergarten, we should be willing to share for the benefit of everyone.

At the same time, we can't give everything to everyone, so we have to set priorities and follow them. This is derogatorily referred to as "rationing." I've got news for you: we ration health care every day in the United States. We never acknowledge this truth or talk about it, though, because most politicians have no knowledge or understanding about health care. 'Rationing' is used either to scare constituents or to accuse opponents of something that sounds vaguely horrible.

I believe that part of our responsibility to each other in a society, especially one built on the promise of life, liberty, and the pursuit of happiness, is to let each other breathe a little easier knowing that if one of us gets hit by a drunk driver and can't work, develops cancer and loses health insurance, or suffers from a mental illness through no fault of our own, we'll be cared for by fellow citizens that have our backs, for whom we are willing to do the same.

It's known as a social contract. It is impossible for every citizen to provide everything they need for themselves, so we should agree to share responsibilities and provide each other with some fundamental human needs, including basic health care.

Politicians hear this type of argument and scream, "Socialism!" End of argument, right? Socialism must be bad, and this sounds like socialism, so instead of having a conversation about what we're trying to accomplish or explaining the problem and debating different strategies to address it, we just stop talking about it.

Medicare is a semi-socialist program. So is Social Security. The VA is a socialist system. Disrupting these programs would be politically risky for any politician, yet so is suggesting expanding access to health care to all Americans. This intellectual dishonesty is a disservice to all of us.

Fortunately, when you're suffering from a true medical emergency, there's a place you can come to be treated whether you're the richest person in the world or don't have a dime to your name: the ER.

CHAPTER TWENTY-EIGHT

My Most Rewarding Case

<u>**Chief complaint: "Chest pain"**</u>

A 42-year-old male presents to the ER by ambulance with a STEMI, or ST-elevation myocardial infarction. A heart attack. Specifically, a heart attack you can see on an ECG (electrocardiogram). ST-elevation refers to a segment on the ECG that can be diagnostic for a heart attack in the right clinical context. When a STEMI comes in by ambulance, every ER worth its salt will have a streamlined process in place to get the patient to a cardiac catheterization lab, or "cath lab," as quickly as possible. Most heart attacks are caused by a blood clot in one or more of the coronary arteries, and as the saying goes, "time is muscle," meaning the faster the clot can be removed and blood flow re-established to the heart muscle, the more heart muscle survives, increasing the odds of the patient recovering with no permanent disability.

Michael was a very cordial, polite man whose demeanor belied his disease process. During a rapid initial evaluation, I discovered a concerning finding. Michael's left arm felt cooler than his right. He had a pulse at his left wrist, but it was weaker than the pulse in his right wrist. I asked the nurse to check his blood pressure in both arms and discovered a difference that was at once concerning and illuminating. His blood pressure was significantly lower in his left arm than his right. At about that time he also said his left arm was starting to feel numb.

Michael wasn't just having a heart attack. Within a few minutes of arrival, it was apparent that he had an aortic dissection, a tear in the aorta, the largest artery in the body. The aorta comes right off the heart and extends all the way down into the abdomen. The right side of your heart pumps blood through your lungs. The left side pumps blood everywhere else in your body, and every drop of it starts in your aorta. There's no such thing as a "little problem" with your aorta.

The late, lovable actor John Ritter reportedly died from an aortic dissection that was initially diagnosed as a heart attack, just like Michael's was thought to be. Anyone who has seen and diagnosed aortic dissections understands how this happens. For starters, the paramedics didn't misinterpret his ECG. His electrocardiogram did in fact show ST-elevation consistent with a heart attack. That's because the aortic root, the part that connects the aorta to your heart, is where your coronary arteries branch off from the aorta to supply blood to your heart. When an aortic dissection extends into your aortic root, it can cut off the blood supply to your heart muscle, and you end up with the same result: a heart attack. Depending on which part of your aorta is involved and how far it extends, the dissection might be managed medically with intensive observation, or you might need emergency surgery.

Arteries have three layers of tissue in their walls. A dissection means that at least two of the layers start to separate or be torn apart. If the tear rips all the way through the blood vessel, in which case the biggest artery in your body starts pumping massive amounts of blood into your chest or belly, you bleed out fairly quickly. If that doesn't sound scary to you, I have failed to adequately describe it, because believe me, it's terrifying.

Bleeding to death isn't the only way you can die from an aortic dissection, though. The aforementioned aortic root also includes your aortic valve which is supposed to keep blood flowing one way—out of your heart and into your aorta. If the valve is disrupted, your heart can't pump blood normally, and blood starts to flow in both directions. This can lead to heart failure, causing fluid to back up into your lungs, which makes it harder to breathe.

Additionally, a dissection can involve other blood vessels, interrupting blood flow to whatever structures those arteries supply—things like your head (which can cause a stroke), your kidneys (which can cause them to fail and put you on dialysis), your stomach and intestines, or an arm or a leg. Michael had decreased blood flow to his left arm because his dissection was stopping blood from flowing normally into his left subclavian artery, which supplies blood to the left arm.

If I haven't been crystal clear on this, let me summarize. Aortic dissections are bad. They scare the crap out of us ER doctors and they kill patients. They can also be extremely tricky to diagnose when their presenting symptoms are more subtle or when masquerading as another serious problem like a heart attack that causes doctors to jump on that issue immediately and waste precious time chasing the wrong problem. Michael was fortunate in one regard: his pale, cool left arm that was becoming numb and in which he had decreased blood pressure immediately told me what the problem was.

I ordered appropriate testing, the mainstay of which is a CT aortogram, where IV contrast is injected during a high-speed CT scan. This confirmed what I already knew. Michael had a type A aortic dissection, meaning it involved his ascending aorta, the part that leaves the heart and travels upward before making a U-turn in your chest and heading downward, becoming the descending aorta. Type A dissections require emergent surgery.

As we worked diligently to diagnose and monitor Michael, his wife arrived. As I saw her at his side, she looked familiar. That was because Janet worked in Housekeeping in the hospital, and while she didn't work primarily in the ER, I had seen her around. I updated Janet on Michael's condition and tried to express my concern without alarming her, all while making arrangements for Michael to be transferred to the closest tertiary care center with cardiothoracic surgery.

When a patient is critically ill and dependent on transfer to another facility to save their life, every minute feels like an hour. Why hasn't the doctor called me back? Why isn't the ambulance here? Why hasn't someone installed a teleportation device like in Star Trek so I could beam him over?

Michael began to complain of feeling short of breath as his wife held his hand. He was talking and remained as courteous and pleasant as ever. I assessed him again, checking his vital signs. After listening to his lungs, one thought crossed my mind.

"Oh. Crap."

Michael's lungs were filling with fluid. He was going into heart failure. His aortic valve wasn't working. His heart muscle wasn't getting enough oxygen. Things were headed straight downhill and fast. I rallied the team to set up for intubation. I had spoken to the thoracic surgeon and the ambulance was on its way.

"Hold on, Michael," I thought. "Don't die in front of your wife right here in the middle of the ER."

The intubation went smoothly, and his oxygen level improved. His blood pressure continued to decrease, though. His only chance at survival was having cardiothoracic surgeons crack open his chest and doing the stuff that cardiothoracic surgeons do.

The ambulance arrived after what seemed like an eternity. Our deeply dedicated staff worked to get him loaded up and out the door as fast as we possibly could. As Michael was wheeled out of the ER and into the ambulance, I was proud of our ER staff for the excellent and very efficient care he received, yet I knew he probably wouldn't make it, and the vision of his sweet wife holding his hand in our ER for maybe the last time ever was too much to think about during a busy shift. I tried to put it out of my head and finish the workday.

At the end of my shift, I looked him up in the EMR (electronic medical record). Nothing there. Probably not a good sign, I concluded before heading home. I didn't sleep well that night. First thing next morning I logged onto the EMR from home. I was pleasantly surprised that I didn't get the dreaded warning, "You are about to enter the record of a deceased patient. Are you sure you want to proceed?" If you ever see that message when you aren't expecting to, it makes you tremble. In Michael's case, I expected it but didn't see it.

I immediately looked for a note from the thoracic surgeon and began reading. "Michael is a 42-year-old male who was transferred for a type A aortic dissection. Patient with ST-elevation on ECG and respiratory failure requiring intubation." The words that followed were chilling. "Patient in cardiac arrest on arrival to the operating room. CPR initiated."

Michael had died. His aortic dissection, as many are, was devastating enough to his heart function and blood flow that he didn't make it. I kept reading.

"Patient placed on heart-lung machine."

Wait. What?

As I read on, the incredible story unfolded. Michael's heart stopped, but that didn't stop the cardiothoracic team. After all, you know what cardiothoracic surgeons and anesthesiologists do day after day? They stop people's hearts, fix them, then restart them. Like mechanics do with an engine—shut it off, take it apart, fix whatever's wrong, then fire it up again and hope you don't end up with any extra parts.

Why let little things like a heart that's not beating and a patient who is technically dead get in the way? The thoracic team worked on Michael for hours, replacing his dissected aorta with a graft and repairing his aortic valve. By no means was Michael out of the woods, but somehow he had made it through the night. I followed his progress from afar day by day until one day Michael was discharged home from the hospital. He actually made it home to his wife and family.

I was in awe of the surgical team. I decided to send them a token of my appreciation, something I've done from time to time throughout my career, though not as often as I should. Being from Toledo, I sent a little something from my hometown: Sweet Hot Pickles and Peppers from a Hungarian restaurant called Tony Packo's. I grew up a huge fan of the television show M*A*S*H. That show is probably part of the reason I became a doctor. While I wanted to be Hawkeye, the character I had a true kinship with was Klinger.

On the show, Klinger hailed from Toledo, undoubtedly because the actor who played Klinger, Jamie Farr, was actually from Toledo. Packo's was mentioned on several episodes of M*A*S*H. I've eaten there many times, but what I love most from Packo's are their Sweet Hot Pickles 'n' Peppers. I'd order them by the case, 12 jars, and would pay almost as much to ship them across the country as the pickles themselves cost, thus they were pretty pricey pickles (say that ten times fast). I've given them to colleagues to convey my appreciation because the pickles mean something to me. Besides, who doesn't like a tasty treat?

I wrote a letter to the cardiothoracic surgery team thanking them for their incredible skill and dedication, and for saving the life of my patient for the sake of his family.

After a few weeks, my thoughts were less consumed by the case. I was content that Michael was alive and well, though on occasion I'd read a progress note from his follow-up visits. Once you become that invested in another human being's life... his very survival... there's a bond between you forever.

Months later, I walked into the ER to start my shift, and was greeted by a gentleman yelling across the ER, "There he is! There's the doctor that saved my life!"

It was Michael, dressed in the uniform of a hospital volunteer. His recovery had gone well. His wife, Janet, still worked at the hospital. Michael was so thankful to those who did everything they could to save his life that he began volunteering at the hospital to pay it back. For years, if we crossed paths during a shift, he would spot me and begin bowing with his arms up in a Wayne's World "We're not worthy" salute, shake my hand and thank me. An ER doctor rarely if ever gets that kind of validation. It felt good every time.

On more than one occasion, Michael mentioned that had he died the day we met, he never would have seen his son graduate, or met his grandchild, or had the time he had cherished with his wife, and that he was thankful for every day of life. It's how we should all live. Michael's remains the most rewarding patient encounter I've ever had.

CHAPTER TWENTY-NINE

Say Something

Chief complaint: Unknown

A 34-year-old male arrived by ambulance. During bedside report, medics stated that he "wouldn't say what's wrong with him." He was writhing in pain. I couldn't get him to open his eyes, and he wouldn't answer any of my questions. He gently rocked from side to side on the gurney, his face contorted as if in agony.

I'd seen patients arrive unable to speak because of severe pain. More often than not, though, they were accompanied by someone who could help provide some clues.

The patient had been in a convenience store when he abruptly dropped to the floor, so 911 was called. He couldn't tell us his name, and we didn't find any identification on him. He became John Doe, born 01/01/1900, as was standard at our facility.

John Doe was an impressively fit, muscular man, just a bit younger than me. I couldn't get him to answer any of my questions. I tried asking yes/no questions that he could shake his head to, but still had no success. His only sounds were grunts and groans.

I'd seen my share of "drama codes" in the ER, when patients demonstrate far more histrionics than are needed for their relatively minor issues. That's not what this was.

Whatever it was, I knew it was bad. I ran through a list of medical conditions that hurt like hell. I considered kidney stone, but even those patients could usually talk to me. I thought about testicular torsion, as that can be awfully painful, but I did a quick exam and found no evidence to support investigating it further. Subarachnoid hemorrhage from a ruptured cerebral aneurysm? That too would be toward the top of the list in terms of sudden onset of intense pain, but those patients don't roll back and forth in bed; they don't want to move at all, because any movement of their head only makes things worse.

The shift was incredibly busy; I really didn't have time to spend *not* talking to a patient, but despite his normal vital signs, his obvious agony demanded the sense of urgency required for patients who were bordering on collapse—patients who were in septic shock, bleeding profusely, or demonstrating symptoms of a heart attack or stroke.

In those first couple of minutes in the ER, he did make one gesture, bringing his fist up to his chest, though his eyes remained squeezed tightly shut as he continued to rock back and forth. Having nothing else to go on, I ordered an ECG and labs. I ordered Dilaudid, a powerful opioid pain medication, to relieve his pain.

I ran through the differential for life-threatening causes of chest pain. Boerhaave syndrome—a rupture of his esophagus? I had actually just seen a case of this a few days prior—an elderly woman who had gone in to have her feeding tube removed. It "snagged" on her esophagus somehow and as it was pulled out her esophagus was ripped open. She had subcutaneous emphysema all over her neck and upper chest. Subcutaneous emphysema is air under the skin. When you press on the skin, it feels like you are crushing Rice Krispies. She had air all over her chest x-ray where it didn't belong. She had bilateral pneumothoraces—both lungs were collapsed. I had to intubate her and place chest tubes on both sides. I checked John Doe for subcutaneous emphysema; he didn't have any.

Pericardial tamponade? Didn't really fit. Myocardial infarction? His ECG and troponin didn't give any indication of it. Tension pneumothorax? There were no other exam findings to support this diagnosis. Pulmonary embolus was always possible and was still fairly high on my list. Given his excruciating pain, though, the diagnosis that came immediately to mind was aortic dissection.

Unlike Michael's presentation, he had no pulse deficit, and his blood pressure was similar in both arms. He was hemodynamically stable, meaning his heart rate, blood pressure, and signs of blood flow throughout his body looked OK.

It felt like time was not on my side, or his, so I ordered a CT angiogram of his chest, and asked the technician to look both at his aorta and for a pulmonary embolus as best she could.

The CT confirmed my worst fear. John Doe had a type A aortic dissection. He needed surgery immediately. While he still couldn't speak despite repeated doses of pain medication, I had no reason to think he couldn't hear me or understand what I told him.

I began telling him what was happening to him and that we needed to transfer him to the tertiary care center twenty-five minutes away when the thoracic surgeon called back. I stepped out of his room to take the call. I relayed the pertinent clinical information to the surgeon, who immediately accepted the patient, and was about to hang up when I heard the nurse yelling from the patient's room.

"He doesn't have a pulse!"

I blurted out, "He's coding," before hanging up the phone and running into his room.

We did the things we do in the emergency room: he was intubated, given fluids, medications, and CPR. It was all to no avail. Unlike Michael's, his heart never beat again.

It was a stark reminder that sometimes the disease process wins out.

John Doe, a young, fit, healthy man, died right in front of me without ever saying a word.

CHAPTER THIRTY

The Unholy Trinity

It's easy to recite the most dramatic or hilarious stories from a career in emergency medicine, but I would be remiss in offering a realistic insider's perspective if I let you think that working in the ER consisted only of heroic efforts to save lives interspersed with humorous encounters.

Being an ER doctor is demanding. It leaves a mark on your soul. The Unholy Trinity of emergency medicine is monotony, uncertainty, and emotional trauma.

Monotony

Believe it or not, most patients with abdominal pain are *not* dying. Abdominal pain can be enormously challenging to diagnose accurately during the first ER visit, sure, but that has more to do with the limitations of testing and the need for time to pass for the clinical picture to clearly emerge.

The approach to abdominal pain is actually pretty straightforward. Get a complete blood count (CBC), basic metabolic panel (BMP), liver function tests (LFTs) and a lipase. Check a urine dip. For women of childbearing age, check a pregnancy test. If there is still any concern, get some imaging—an ultrasound to look for gallstones or an ovarian cyst or torsion, a CT to look for most other diagnoses. We do this several times every shift, and thousands of times over the course of a career. It becomes routine.

After you've incised and drained a few hundred abscesses on heroin users, the next one is hard to get excited about. You might still tell a colleague about how bad one smelled or how much pus came out, but otherwise cutting into an abscess is about as monotonous as emergency medicine gets. I've seen videos on YouTube of popping a zit or squeezing a small abscess and wondered how many hits I would get if I were able to upload a video of one of my patients' abscesses that drained so much pus that we needed suction. Damn you, HIPAA!

Like any learned skill, once you've done it day after day, year after year, what thrilled you the first time you did it becomes tedious.

Uncertainty

Throughout virtually every minute spent on shift in the ER, there is a baseline anxiety over what might come through the door next. Being in a constant state of alert exacts a physical and mental toll. Shifts are frequently draining, primarily because of the question lingering over every patient encounter: "What am I missing?"

There is nothing more reassuring than having complete confidence that you know exactly what's wrong with the patient and what to do about it.

For my money, the most satisfying diagnosis in emergency medicine is the nursemaid's elbow. A father playing with his daughter grabs her arm and twirls her around as she giggles. Suddenly, the toddler screams out. Dad might even hear or feel a pop and is certain he's dislocated or broken something. The parents scoop up the child and rush to the ER. The registration clerk enters a chief complaint, "Won't move arm," and I am instantly relieved. When the nurse writes in his note, "Father was swinging child around while playing. Now child won't move left arm," I am 95% sure I know what's wrong: the child has a nursemaid's elbow.

I immediately go to the patient's bedside. I know the parents are freaked out. I understand that the child is in pain. I am confident I will make all of them feel better.

After listening to how it happened, confirming my suspicion as to what's wrong, I give them my spiel.

"There are two bones in the forearm: the radius, which goes down the thumb side, and the ulna. In toddlers, the end of the radius is loosely held in place at the elbow by a ligament that is not yet fully developed. Any motion that tugs straight out on the arm can partially pull it out of place; it's called a subluxation—it's not a dislocation or a broken bone. You end up with what you have noticed— she cries and refuses to move her arm."

The parents figured she broke her wrist or dislocated something, so hearing that it's neither of those starts to calm them.

I continue explaining, "I need to perform a maneuver that she won't like but which is very fast." I specifically avoid saying "it will hurt" because the child is injured, not dumb, and if she hears that it will be painful, I will have to contend with a less cooperative patient.

I maneuver her arm a bit, she cries, I tell the parents that I'm done and am pretty sure the problem is fixed and that I will check back shortly, then I leave the room.

Her parents are initially skeptical. Don't we need x-rays? How do I know that's what's wrong? Wasn't her wrist the problem, not her elbow? How do I know it's fixed?

Within a few minutes, the parents notice she is moving her arm around like there was never anything wrong. The patient's arm was completely disabled, and without any testing whatsoever I made a clinical diagnosis based solely on my study and understanding of medicine, then I performed a procedure to completely fix the problem and relieve the patient's pain. The parents are incredulous and grateful. It just doesn't get any better than that in medicine.

If only every ER patient was that straightforward. Most are not, and it is the uncertainty that keeps us on edge every minute we're working. When a parent frantically rushes through the ER entrance carrying a child, our minds start racing. We run through a list in our heads.

"Is the child seizing? Is he in status epilepticus? What dose of Ativan do I want to give? Will the nurses be able to get an IV? I better give intranasal midazolam. Does he have altered mental status? Meningitis? If so, I want the LP tray at the bedside now, and I need to order antibiotics STAT so they can be started as soon as I finish the lumbar puncture. Is he short of breath? I wonder if he has a congenital heart defect. What are the cyanotic heart lesions again? The 5 T's: Tetralogy of Fallot, total anomalous venous return, tricuspid atresia, truncus arteriosus and transposition of the great vessels. Yes! That's it! God, I hope it's not one of those. If so, I better call pediatric cardiology right now. Or maybe he got into something. Don't forget to ask what medications are in the home."

The list goes on. When the chief complaint pops up on the tracker, "Nursemaid's elbow," you breathe a sigh of relief.

Emotional Trauma

A 28-year-old woman presents 13 weeks pregnant because she has had some spotting and cramping. She is tearful and anxious because this is her third pregnancy, the first two having ended in miscarriage, and she and her husband have been trying to have a baby for two years. She fears she is having another miscarriage.

The medical decision-making is easy. Her vitals are stable; her abdomen is benign. Check a hematocrit, look for her Rh from a previous visit or order one, get a quantitative hCG and an ultrasound. Couldn't be simpler. Move on to the next patient and manage your other patients until her results are back.

Her ultrasound shows fetal demise. No ectopic pregnancy—nothing else to do except tell her.

I enter the room, grab the rolling stool, and take a seat next to her. She and her husband already deduced there was a problem when the ultrasound tech didn't show them the baby's heartbeat, but they're waiting to hear it from me. I might start by explaining the rest of her results or asking about her pain level, but eventually there's no escaping the elephant in the room.

"Mrs. and Mr. Silverstein, I'm sorry to tell you this, but your ultrasound showed that you have had a miscarriage."

I let it sink in for a moment. She begins to sob. His eyes well up with tears as he holds her hand more tightly. For me, the medicine was the easy part, having done it so many times. From the standpoint of degree of difficulty, vaginal bleeding in the first trimester of pregnancy falls lower on the uncertainty scale, higher on the monotony scale.

For Mrs. and Mr. Silverstein, they've just found out that their unborn child is dead. What they've wanted and dreamed about for the past two years, a shared devotion made of parts of both of them, a bundle of joy to love and protect, has once again been taken from them. Their devastation and grief are raw, and I have no choice but to share their emotions, because that's what human beings with empathy do.

Perhaps later in that shift, I have to tell a patient that he has metastatic cancer. A woman who was violently raped has just been put in room 7. I need to obtain the details of what happened to her and live with them in my head, knowing what one fellow human being is capable of doing to another. Another patient is brought in by ambulance after a suicide attempt. A drunk driver is in the ER with police. While we don't confront death on every ER shift, each shift does put us face to face with our collective flaws, weaknesses, vices, and cruelty toward one another.

At one point my hospital was building a new ER and I was fortunate enough to participate in the design process. I asked for metal detector. I was told we didn't need one, that a metal detector would be "unwelcoming." Our sister hospital had one, and their Chief of Security came to a meeting, at my invitation, to inform those present of the hundreds of knives and dozens of guns they'd taken off patients and visitors since obtaining their metal detector.

I tried to build a case for a metal detector based on logic and facts. I found online prison rolls and was able to verify that many of the offenders had been treated in our ER within the past year. I randomly looked up some higher profile criminals in the community, including a rapist and someone who had murdered police—they'd been patients, too. It made perfect sense to me. Violent criminals are less likely to have private insurance and primary care providers. Where do you think they go when they need medical care?

We didn't get a metal detector. Having one would seem "accusatory" or "set the wrong tone" toward patients and visitors, or so they said. We all knew the truth: metal detectors cost more money, and it was not deemed worth the cost to offer additional protection to the patients and staff inside the ER.

Abuses that are never tolerated elsewhere are typically treated as an expected part of the job in the ER. If someone assaults a police officer, his sentence is often harsher than if he'd attacked a random citizen. If someone assaults a health care worker, do you know what happens more often than not? Nothing. A 15-year-old once spit directly in my face. Far too many patients have tried to bite, scratch, grab or punch me. I've known several coworkers who were injured during an assault at work.

Emotional trauma is cumulative over the course of one's career. We are often bored, anxious, skeptical, untrusting, frustrated with the EMR and alarm-fatigued, not to mention hungry and thirsty, all in the same day. We experience these negative emotions repeatedly, which over time robs us of a bit of our humanity. This explains why most of us who work in the ER share a dark, cynical sense of humor that would shock or disgust the uninitiated. It's a necessary defense mechanism. It becomes difficult to look at people the same way. We're often accused of being burnt out. I think many of us look at the rest of you as naïve and unaware.

Who would put up with working conditions such as these, and why?

We do, because relieving pain, providing comfort, solving problems, diagnosing and treating illness and injury and saving lives are worth doing. The noblest act of which humans are capable is to sacrifice in the service of others. You take the good with the bad because both are part of life. I've done my share of complaining about my job, but the truth is that if I had to do it all over again, I can't picture myself doing anything else.

CHAPTER THIRTY-ONE

What a Perceptive Little Girl

I slid the glass door to the left, then drew back the curtain to enter the room of my next patient, an adorable four-year-old girl in a pink dress with white polka dots, her hair in a ponytail. As I started to introduce myself, her big brown eyes lit up, and she began almost dancing. I couldn't help but take note of her reaction, wondering what she was so excited about, as young children often respond to my presence by crying or cowering behind their parents.

Her little feet couldn't hold still as she practically jumped up and down next to her dad. She pulled his shirt toward her and cupped her hand over his ear to whisper something to him. He chuckled, then whispered back to her so that I could hear, "Why don't you ask him?"

She folded her hands together and bravely took a step forward, looking up directly into my eyes and smiled as she asked me, "Are you Mr. Incredible?"

I laughed, wishing that were the case, but that didn't stop me from smiling as I sucked in my gut and puffed out my chest for the rest of the day.

CHAPTER THIRTY-TWO

A Place to Put Your Junk

Every ER doctor in the country has her or his stories that involve people putting stuff where it doesn't belong or doing things to themselves most of us wouldn't think to do. I feel obligated to share some of them. These are the stories I often *pull out* at parties. Those of us who don't live life so close to the edge seem to enjoy the salacious details of those who do, especially when things don't go as planned. Without further ado, here is a smattering of some of the most colorful tales.

Get Out of Jail Free Card

Prisoners will go to extraordinary lengths to buy themselves a few hours outside their cells. I once saw a woman from prison who got her hands on a ball point pen, took the ink cartridge out of the center of it, stabbed herself in the right thigh with it, then proceeded to snap it off so the lower half couldn't be pulled out. I x-rayed it, confirmed it was there, numbed the area up with some local anesthetic, made an incision, located it with some forceps and pulled it out.

I've also seen prisoners who swallowed items that were not meant to be digested. One guy swallowed four AA batteries, though the joke was on him, because you don't really have to do anything about those, so he immediately went back to jail.

Another guy swallowed a handful of metal bedsprings. Because of the number of them and their unusual shape, he underwent endoscopic removal of the springs by a gastroenterologist.

I imagine in jail you have a lot of time on your hands, and if men have enough time, eventually something else ends up in their hands. I saw a 20-something male who literally broke his dick. Yes, it is actually possible to fracture your penis: a broken boner. The structures that fill with blood to give a man an erection, called corpora cavernosa (which is the plural—corpus cavernosum is the singular form) can break, causing significant bleeding into the soft tissue of the penis, causing it to swell to several times its normal size, but not in a good way. A urologist has to repair it surgically. All those times my Drill Sergeants called us "brokedicks" I had no idea that was a real thing.

A Proud Father

A fifteen-year-old boy comes to the ER claiming, "I put a sewing needle in my dick." He'd taken a two-inch long sewing needle and slid it inside his urethra until it disappeared. X-rays showed it to be at the level of his prostate. No way that was coming back out. His father looked like the prototypical business executive, dressed in a nice suit, hair perfectly coiffed—the picture of success. You could feel the humiliation and quiet rage in the room. A urology consult and trip to the operating room just made things worse. Kids…

Hick Farms

A 46-year-old man complains of "having a summer sausage in my butt." A Hickory Farms gift pack always made a nice Christmas gift. I had bought them as gifts myself in the past, yet for some reason I was picturing the pack with the small single-size servings of sausage and

186

cheese. After establishing that this incident occurred while he and his wife were being "adventurous," I asked him how big the aforementioned summer sausage was, roughly. He held his hands apart at a distance far greater than I had anticipated, along the lines of a foot and half. "The whole thing just disappeared," he explained, and he hadn't seen any sign of it since. It was nothing a trip to the GI suite couldn't fix.

Odds in Ends

A 67-year-old woman complains of having a vibrator in her rectum. What bothered her most was the fact that it was still running. Curious, I laid my hand on her belly in the left lower quadrant. Yep, still running. Using a vaginal speculum in her rectum and a pair of long forceps, I was able to retrieve it.

From time to time every ER doc pulls a dildo or vibrator out—"the one that got away." I once removed a 15-inch double-ended purple jelly dong that the ER staff affectionately nicknamed "The Purple People Eater".

Our base station once got a call from medics in the field who picked up a patient with a vibrator in his butt that was still running. They wanted to know if they could bring the patient to us or whether they should go to a Trauma Center. Only in an ER would staff hear that complaint and look at each other matter-of-factly and say, "Doesn't sound traumatic. Bring it here."

On July 4th, a 52-year-old guy comes in "because I have a bingo dauber stuck in my butt." Not a huge bingo player, I asked him what a bingo dauber was. He explained that it was a bottle filled with ink that one used to mark off the numbers on bingo cards. It was about the size of a small bottle of shampoo. Sure enough, when I used a vaginal speculum to look in his butt, the bottom end of said bottle was exactly what I saw. I sedated him and tried to extract the bottle, which didn't want to budge. I ended up using a tenaculum, an instrument with two pointy metal teeth at the end. I had to grab the bottle along the bottom edge, puncturing the side and the bottom of the bottle with the two teeth, which gave me something solid to grab, and I was able to slowly back it out. Given that the dauber was filled with blue ink, the fluid began to leak out once I pierced two holes in it. The entire procedure was slightly traumatic, thus he had some minor oozing of blood from the mucosa inside his rectum. He was a White guy. I couldn't resist pointing out the combination to the nurses and techs in the room. "Red, white and blue! Happy 4th of July!"

Nuts and Bolts

A 34-year-old man presents to the ER after he tried to use a metal washer as a "cock ring." I apologize for the crude language, but I figure if you're still reading this book, you might not be terribly offended if I explain how a grown man decided to use a relatively small metal washer as a cock ring.

I am sure there was a time before entering my horizon-expanding chosen profession when I didn't have a clue what a cock ring was or did. In case you too are uninitiated, a cock ring is a ring that is placed around the base of the penis and sometimes the testicles to provide gentle constriction, theoretically to maintain engorgement with blood, giving the man a harder, bigger erection. They are usually made of flexible materials like silicone or rubber.

This guy decided to use a metal washer that was maybe one inch in internal diameter. He must have had a hell of a time getting his penis through it in the first place, but he managed. The constriction did indeed impede blood flow back from the penis, resulting in impressive enlargement. It was not exactly hard, though, and I have no idea what he could have used it for, but one thing was certain: it wasn't coming off.

Imagine if you will a normal sized penis constricted down to 1 inch at the base and having a diameter of what appeared to be 3 inches beyond the metal washer. The risk of this is that it eventually stops blood flow to the penis completely and can result in the penis dying—something both doctors and every man on the planet refer to as *not good*.

The only way to remove it was to cut it off (the washer, that is). Fortunately, using a ring saw, pliers and some elbow grease, I was able to cut through and snap the washer in two places to remove it. YOLO.

Tow Be or Not Tow Be

A 49-year-old man presents having put *his* junk where it didn't belong and didn't fit, this time using a metal tow hook instead of a washer.

I can't explain what a tow hook does as sophomorically as I can giggle about a cock ring, but this was far more impressive. A metal tow hook is typically fastened at the end of heavy strapping or a metal cable, such as on a winch, to pull something heavy like a car. There is a stout metal ring with a protruding hook to grab onto whatever is being towed. This was no washer; this thing was solid!

I tried the ring saw but it didn't even make a scratch in the tow hook. I inquired about what kind of tool orthopedic surgeons use to cut the hardware they use for joint replacements or internal fixations but couldn't get my hands on anything.

Most ERs have a toolbox stashed somewhere. I know it sounds like I must be using medical slang and that by "toolbox" you think I am referring to a procedure cart that contains specialized medical equipment. I am not. I am talking about a toolbox. It's never a good thing if you need your doctor to grab the toolbox. It might indicate you've buried a fishhook in your finger, and we need to grab the wire cutters and pliers from the toolbox to remove it. Or you shot yourself with a nail gun, and we use the pliers to pull the nail out of your kneecap. It's not like we use a rusty set of old tools, but they're not exactly precision-crafted surgical instruments, either.

It turns out that if you stick your dick through a tow hook and wait until it triples in size before coming into the ER, there isn't even anything in the toolbox that will get the job done. This is where the improvisational and problem-solving skills of a highly trained emergency physician come into play.

By that, I mean the only idea I could come up with was to use bolt cutters. Not a small pair of bolt cutters, mind you. A pair of BFBC. I sedated the patient, mostly so he wouldn't have to see the excitement or the fear on my face or hear what we might say throughout the procedure. Besides, if the worse-case scenario happened, and I ended up slipping with the bolt cutters and snapping his dick off, I wanted a few minutes to think about how I would tell him when he woke up.

The problem was, even after squeezing the long handles of the bolt cutters together as hard as I could until sweat was running down my face, I made zero progress. I needed backup. I asked for someone to grab Cody to come to the room.

Cody was an ER tech; one who happened to have played offensive line for the Chicago Bears. His NFL career was short, but the guy had actually been on Soldier Field as an O-lineman in a Bears uniform. I stand 6-foot-2, and Cody made me look small, not to mention glad that I never played defensive line for the Lions.

With Cody on one side, pulling one long handle of the bolt cutters toward him with all his might, and me on the opposite side doing the same, we pulled until we heard an incredibly loud "SNAP". I was afraid to look down. When I did, I was rewarded with the sight of the metal tow hook still tightly squeezing the patient's abnormally engorged penis. I had slid a metal spatula between the tow hook and his penis to protect the skin, and it had worked.

A metal ring doesn't fall off or open up when you cut one side, however. You have to make two cuts, which meant we had to do the same thing on the opposite side of the ring. We repeated our efforts, sweating profusely before the terrifying yet satisfying SNAP echoed in the room once again.

This time when I looked down, I was thrilled to see that the metal tow hook was lying in his lap in two pieces, with his misshapen but still intact penis right where I'd left it.

Sometimes this job is just plain fun.

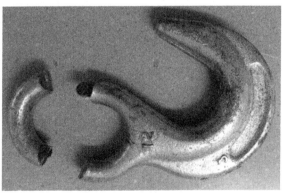

The actual tow hook

CHAPTER THIRTY-THREE

The Wrong Stuff

Your butt isn't the only portal of entry for stuff that doesn't belong in your body. Plenty of people put things in their bodies that they shouldn't the old-fashioned way—by swallowing them.

Every medical specialty has its own particular skill set. Urologists are experts at performing surgery on the genitourinary tract, fixing everything from bladder incontinence, testicular torsion and kidney stones to prostate surgery and nephrectomy. Endocrinologists treat all manner of, well, endocrine problems, including diabetes, thyroid disorders and a host of other conditions most of us have to look up. Rheumatologists investigate patients with bizarre, seemingly unrelated symptoms that stump the rest of us in addition to managing autoimmune and related conditions. The list goes on.

Our expertise in the ER encompasses the medical and surgical emergencies of each specialty. We are experts at identifying a broad range of maladies and assessing how serious they might be. Most patients sick enough to require admission to the hospital come through the ER.

If our specialty is on the cutting edge of any aspect of medicine, it is being the first to witness the adverse medical consequences of inventive new trends in self-destruction. Examples include the "Tide pod challenge," "cinnamon challenge" and "hot water challenge," to name a few.

The entire purpose of the medical profession is to stymie natural selection—to keep those alive who otherwise might be too weak, sick, or stupid to survive. Modern medicine allows for the "survival of the unfittest." It's expensive, of course, and some may question whether it hurts or helps humanity in the long run, but it's what we do.

Before the trends become established, however, the "challenge" for doctors is trying to figure out what the hell you took before you passed out and were found unconscious, prompting someone to call 911 to send you to us.

A 46-year-old veterinarian was brought to the ER by ambulance after he was found unresponsive. His eyes were open, but he couldn't talk. Was he having a stroke? He had no other findings to suggest so. It had to be toxicologic, but his urine drug screen was negative. He improved over the next hour and was able to sheepishly tell me he had injected himself with ketamine, which he had access to because it was used to sedate animals. Not long after, ketamine was in vogue as a recreational drug, affectionately nicknamed "Special K."

"Awesome," I thought to myself. "We should name all drugs after breakfast cereals."

"Tired of the same old bitter heroin? Try new Kellogg Sugar Smack!"

A confused 38-year-old woman arrives by ambulance with low blood pressure and a funky heart rhythm on ECG. I couldn't tell what the rhythm was, and the odd morphologies of her various QRS complexes made no sense to me. I decided to consult the cardiologist to help me determine what was going on with her heart.

When an ER doctor consults a specialist, we usually know exactly what needs to be done. Maybe I've diagnosed a peritonsillar abscess and am consulting an ENT for follow-up or emergent drainage of the abscess. Or I've diagnosed appendicitis and am consulting a surgeon to take the patient to the operating room. That kind of thing.

Less frequent are calls to consultants because we fear we are missing something, or because the pieces don't add up to anything that makes sense to us, so we're looking for help. When I make those calls, I'm always afraid the consultant will quickly respond with the correct answer as though it should have been obvious, and I... no, make that both of us... will think I'm an idiot.

But that's not usually what happens. If a patient is in the ER with some bizarre presentation that leaves me stumped despite two decades of experience seeing tens of thousands of patients, the consultant is often at a loss as well. In the case of my patient's ECG, I seem to recall the cardiologist's response upon reviewing the ECG being, "What am I supposed to do with that?"

I laughed, because that was exactly what I was wondering! Since I had managed to bring the patient's blood pressure up to an acceptable level, we both agreed that the best thing to do, contrary to Teddy Roosevelt's advice, was nothing.

Once her husband arrived in the ER, I was able to obtain information from him that explained her presentation. She had been trying to wean herself off oxycodone, a potent opioid, so she was consuming up to four boxes of Imodium, an anti-diarrheal medication, every day for the past two weeks. It hadn't been on my radar at that time, but sure enough, within a couple of months there were more frequent reports about Imodium being used as a recreational drug.

A 33-year-old bodybuilder presents with altered mental status, but his urine drug screen was negative. I worked him up to the hilt, including a CT and lumbar puncture, which did show a small but abnormal number of white blood cells. I tentatively pursued a diagnosis of encephalitis until he became completely coherent again, at which time he was able to tell me he'd done GHB, gamma-hydroxybutyrate, which I learned had become a popular drug in the weightlifting community. GHB is also used as a date rape drug.

A 68-year-old woman presented to the ER by ambulance as a "Code Stroke" due to aphasia—an inability to speak. She looked right at me but didn't say a word. She had no facial droop and moved her arms and legs symmetrically with good strength. I'd seen strokes with aphasia as the only presenting symptom before, so I took it quite seriously and worked her up for a stroke. Her symptoms began to resolve. When stroke-like symptoms resolve quickly, such a presentation becomes diagnosable as a TIA, a transient ischemic attack, or "mini-stroke" as it is sometimes called.

She was unable to provide any other information while in the ER. Her daughter showed up once the patient was on the medical floor, and after talking to her mother, she realized what had happened and informed the hospitalist. The patient was visiting her daughter from out of state and had eaten some cookies that were in the freezer. Turns out they were marijuana cookies, and the patient wasn't having a stroke; she was just high.

An 18-year-old boy presents after his mother found him not breathing and blue on his bedroom floor. She called 911, and EMS gave him naloxone (Narcan). The patient was awake, alert and breathing upon arrival. He said he had a job interview the next day and was very nervous about it, so he borrowed some medicine from a friend to help him sleep. The medication was Oxydose, a liquid form of oxycodone. I hadn't heard of that specific formulation despite the fact that I was well-versed with opioid overdoses. His friend had been prescribed Oxydose due to chronic pain from orthopedic surgery. Oxydose contained 20 mg of oxycodone in 1 mL of solution. The patient said he'd taken a "swig" of the liquid, or a mouthful. An average swallow probably downs about 20 mL of liquid, which means this patient ingested up to 400 mg of oxycodone, or the equivalent of 80 Percocet tablets. For an opioid-naïve patient, you know what that does to you? It makes you apneic! You stop breathing and turn blue, just as his mother found him. In trying to calm himself down and get some sleep before his big job interview, he nearly killed himself.

CHAPTER THIRTY-FOUR

Covid-19

Fear. Rage. Those are the two dominant emotions for me and many other ER docs since the onset of the Covid-19 pandemic. Fear came first.

I live and practice in the Seattle area, the first epicenter of the crisis in the U.S., with the hardest-hit ER in the early days of the pandemic being just down the road from my own. On February 29, 2020, the first U.S. death from Covid-19 was reported here in Washington, and we instantly found ourselves in crisis management mode in a national tragedy that to this point has continued unabated.

At the time the pandemic began claiming lives in the United States, we knew almost nothing about Covid-19 except that it was easily spread and was far deadlier than influenza. Every waking moment of every day was spent either working in the ER or trying to figure out how to keep ourselves and our families safe.

Some doctors moved out of their homes to avoid bringing the virus home and killing their loved ones. Doctors improvised their routines to mitigate their risk as best they could: come home, strip at the door, put their clothes immediately into the washing machine, then shower. Avoid hugging their spouses and kids when they worked and for several days afterward to try to ensure they wouldn't spread it. Update their wills. Get their affairs in order. Tell people they love them. Finish a book that's been on the back burner for far too long.

At first, I must admit that I was foolish enough to think that the management of the Covid-19 pandemic, unlike other threats we faced in recent years, would be grounded in science and managed by scientists and physicians. Covid-19 couldn't be political because this was medicine, and medicine deals with facts and reality. It was apparent early on that this reality was going to be harsh, which also meant that it could not be denied.

I was dead wrong. We, as a nation, allowed politicization of a virus because we looked to politicians for answers rather than scientists and doctors. With regard to Covid-19, conspiracy theories and denial have ruled the day, but only one reality exists: Donald J. Trump is personally responsible for the deaths of tens, if not hundreds, of thousands of Americans. I don't know how anyone could look at the facts and reach any other conclusion.

As a doctor, if I willfully ignored the best evidence available, disregarded standards of care, dismissed the expertise of my colleagues, and recklessly advised a patient to take a course of action that directly led to his or her death, I'd be sued. If I did it to three or four patients, I would lose my medical license. A few more patients harmed in this manner, and I would very likely be criminally charged with negligent homicide, manslaughter, or perhaps second-degree murder.

Yet when our elected and appointed "leaders" ignore facts and spread dangerous disinformation, they are never held to account.

Perhaps the gravest threat to democracies across the world is, as Tom Nichols so brilliantly wrote, *The Death of Expertise*. Our national leadership shunned and ridiculed the experts. We listened to the loudest voices rather than the smartest ones. Our recent years, perhaps decades, of intellectual dishonesty and celebration of ignorance caught up with us quickly.

Early on, we needed to know whether the virus was airborne or spread by droplets so that we would know whether we needed N95 masks, for example. Credible experts and reliable accounts indicated that it was airborne, which meant we should have been using N95 masks at a minimum in all cases. Many doctors argued with their own hospital administrations about this point. Some were even fired.

Well, Donald Trump knew. I heard him say it on the Woodward tapes. Fortunately, the ER doctors I work with were smart enough to act based on their own assessment of the risk and the science rather than deferring to those giving wrong information and bad guidance, even when the erroneous or malicious instruction was coming from their own organizations or the CDC.

After Donald Trump called hydroxychloroquine "one of the biggest game changers in the history of medicine," one of his followers unintentionally killed himself by ingesting it. At the time Trump uttered the words, science hadn't yet determined whether hydroxychloroquine helped or not. That's what made it so dangerous. As it turns out, hydroxychloroquine doesn't work against Covid-19. Trump was wrong.

He called Covid-19 a hoax. Wrong.

He said anyone who wanted a test could get one. Wrong.

Trump said convalescent plasma was "a historic breakthrough." Wrong.

He claimed it was like seasonal flu. Wrong. That it affected "virtually nobody." Wrong.

He said it would magically disappear. Wrong. That it would go away with the heat of summer. Wrong.

Then he alleged that it would disappear after the election, as if thousands of Americans were dying every day to score political points. Wrong.

Trump proposed injecting bleach, or using light "inside the body," both of which are blatantly idiotic. He later tried to say he was joking, but again, I heard him say it.

Why did anyone take the word of a willfully ignorant serial liar about a medical matter? Why? I really want to know. Why would anyone dismiss Dr. Anthony Fauci, a lifelong public servant with specialized training in infectious disease and public health, in favor of a know-nothing blowhard who they heard talk about downplaying the virus with their own ears?

In case you haven't caught on, the fear of the early days yielded to the primary emotion of rage: rage against the idiocy of listening to the twice-impeached, two-time loser of the popular vote Donald J. Trump dismissing science and facts. Trump wasn't good at casinos, steaks, universities, marriage, foundations, airlines, fidelity to things like vows and oaths, water, vodka or governing, among others, so why did a single American take his word about any health care-related matter?

On top of it all, not only did Trump not lift a finger to help, not only did he dismiss the science and ignore the reality of the pandemic—he went a step further. When we didn't have enough PPE to keep ourselves safe, what did Trump do? He accused health care workers of stealing it and selling it out the back door of the hospital. As the death toll began to skyrocket, what did he do? He accused doctors of fraudulently inflating the death counts to make more money.

We didn't need a President who "showed confidence." We needed a President who demonstrated competence. We didn't have one. Because of Donald

Trump's gross negligence and outright stupidity, far too many Americans paid the ultimate price.

While it was known that large gatherings were superspreader events, Trump held as many rallies as he could, often ignoring local guidelines, killing some of his own constituents while exhibiting a pathologic disregard for human life.

When he got Covid-19 himself, Trump didn't rely on hydroxychloroquine, did he? No, he got monoclonal antibodies, which have proven effective in reducing disease severity and mortality.

Nor did he make even the slightest effort to protect others. Rather, he went for a joyride, needlessly exposing Secret Service agents to the potentially lethal disease.

If Trump wants to take credit for the vaccine, perhaps some credit is in order, though I would think that a true conservative might point out that it was capitalism that drove the vaccine timeline, not government intervention.

Pfizer, which did not accept government funds to develop its vaccine in collaboration with BioNTech, and the other pharmaceutical companies were *always* going to get a vaccine to market as quickly as possible.

For someone who has desperately craved credit, Trump hasn't exactly been a champion of vaccination. Rather than using the occasion to encourage Americans to follow suit, he got his shot in secret. Then again, courage and leadership have never been Trump's strong suits, which explains why former Presidents Clinton, Bush and Obama were invited to participate in an ad campaign to implore all Americans to get vaccinated, while Trump was excluded.

Look at the dramatic drop in new Covid-19 cases and deaths as a result of vaccination and consider what might have been possible had Donald Trump been a fierce advocate for wearing masks, social distancing, and avoiding gatherings even for one year. Tens of thousands of Americans would still be alive.

It is a national tragedy that so many people have been unwilling to make even the smallest, most inconsequential sacrifices to protect all of us. We aren't needing to seek shelter in basements as bombs are dropped on us night after night as the people of London did during World War II. I fear for this country if this is the best we can do in a time of crisis. Those of us in the ER and elsewhere in the hospital are risking our lives to care for patients, yet so many others aren't willing to cover their mouths and noses with a piece of cloth, all because their hero thinks it is weak to do so.

The economic devastation brought on by Covid-19 is heartbreaking. All of our energy should be spent on how we get through this together, yet we can't agree on the most basic facts, or make the simplest of shared sacrifices for each other.

I am proud and inspired, however, because that's not what I see at work every day. Despite the fear, not a single ER doctor I know wavered one bit in their dedication to treating every patient who came through the doors. That's the definition of courage—withstanding fear and danger to persevere in their mission.

Like most crises, Covid-19 has brought out the best and worst of humanity. Rather than be disillusioned about the worst of us, I choose to be inspired by the best of us. I can think of none better than the women and men who work, day-in and day-out, to care for those at their time of greatest need.

CHAPTER THIRTY-FIVE

A Love Letter to the ER

To everyone I've ever worked with, the HUCs, techs, ER nurses and doctors who work 24/7 to care for the nation's sickest and most vulnerable patients, I want to tell you how much I respect, admire, and appreciate you.

I've said many times to many people that when it comes to emergency medicine, no one else gets it. Unless you've worked in an ER for some period of time or are married to someone who does, you'll never understand. My wife gets it, because she's heard me talk about it for two and a half decades. "Normal" people don't get it. Physicians and nurses who work everywhere else in the hospital or in health care don't understand. Every time I've ever sat in a conference room in a meeting with someone who doesn't come from the ER, it's been obvious that they don't have the first clue about what we do every day.

But I do. I get it. Every aspect of it. Every in and out of what your jobs require. Every nuance.

This book is a compendium of anecdotes I've written down over the course of my career, mainly because I didn't want to forget relevant details. A career's worth of stories from the ER affects your life in ways big and small.

For starters, you've never seen a more baby-proofed house than mine when my children were young. I've never owned a coffee table—I've seen way too many kids split their heads open falling into them. Every drawer or cabinet that contained something sharp or poisonous had a lock on it. Every jagged surface had padding on it.

We owned a cabin with a beautiful stone hearth exposing a jagged rock edge that stood about a foot and a half off the ground. We placed foam padding all the way around it. Years after selling it, I rented the cabin for a writer's retreat, and was amused and comforted to see that the foam padding was still in place. At least I wasn't the only paranoid parent out there.

After one of my partners pronounced a child dead who had asphyxiated while reaching into a toy box, I went home, dumped the toys on the floor, threw away the rigid toy box in favor of one with collapsible sides, and never again cared if the floor was messy.

I grew up riding dirt bikes. When my boys were about 6 and 9, we bought them ATVs and all their riding gear. The first time I took them to sand dunes to learn to ride, a lunatic going about 60 mph through the sandy parking area on a dune buggy missed my younger son by about five feet. Later, my wife and I heard the story of friends of friends whose teenager flipped over his UTV and died. After that, all I could picture was one of my kids zooming down the street by our cabin and hitting the irrigation ditch on the side of the road and flipping over. I sold them.

That's not to say I think you can make life risk-free, nor should you try. Being an ER doctor makes you aware of lurking dangers, though, sometimes to the point of being fearful, I suppose. Overall, I just try to be smart and not take foolish chances that would later lead to kicking myself, thinking, "Why didn't I see it coming?"

At some point, being an emergency physician ceases to just be your job. It's part and parcel of who you are. By my rough calculations, I have treated over 50,000 ER patients in my career and counting. That's a solid number. I've written of some encounters that went as well as anyone could have hoped, and some that didn't. It wouldn't have been particularly interesting to read about tens of thousands of cases that went as expected, which says a lot about what it means to be an ER doc.

I didn't tell you about all the heart attack patients we quickly diagnosed and whisked off to the cath lab in 20 minutes; the GI bleeders we transfused, reversed their anticoagulation, fluid-resuscitated, intubated and admitted to the ICU for emergent endoscopy; the patients in septic shock who got a central line, fluids, antibiotics and pressors; the patients with a ruptured abdominal aortic aneurysm we quickly diagnosed with bedside ultrasound and sent to the operating room where the vascular surgeon saved their lives; the dangerous overdoses that were quickly identified and treated to prevent cardiovascular collapse; all kinds of true emergencies; even finding some zebras among the horses.

24/7, on nights, weekends, and holidays, ER doctors, nurses and staff stand ready to help anyone who comes in the door, regardless of their ability to pay. I remain inspired by those who sacrifice so much to serve others. I am humbled to count myself among them and remain grateful for the privilege of being involved in the lives of so many people in some small way.

I want to acknowledge and thank everyone outside the ER who make emergency medicine work. A patient in a high-speed motor vehicle collision who ruptures his liver would die if not for the incredible skill and expertise of a trauma surgeon. Emergency physicians don't perform emergent appendectomies or stop a patient with an ectopic pregnancy from bleeding to death. We aren't the ones who care for patients in the hospital day in and day out. Our friends and colleagues, the hospitalists, intensivists, and specialists do that. Emergency medicine is a team sport. ER doctors work closely with other highly skilled physicians and the vast resources of the hospital to save lives. I am grateful to know and work with all of them.

I must also express my sincere appreciation for all departments in the hospital on whom the ER relies so heavily. Considering the fact that an ER might be asked to solve almost any problem imaginable at any time of the day or night, the army of professionals required to address virtually any health care crisis is formidable to say the least. The emergency department is incredibly dependent on a large cadre of highly skilled experts: social workers, respiratory therapists, pharmacists, registration, laboratory services, vascular technicians, and the entire radiology department. Thank you all!

I need to give special recognition, though, to those who work in the ER.

To all the health unit coordinators, or "HUCs," I don't even know how to begin to describe your jobs to outsiders. Think of being an air traffic controller if the skies were filled with random flights headed every which direction being flown by drunk pilots while the phone rings off the hook, crazy people scream, and alarms blare in the background. As an ER doctor, I pride myself on my ability to multitask, but HUCs make multitasking an artform. No ER functions without do-it-all HUCs. The proof lies in the panicked look on an ER doctor's face at 3 a.m. when they look around and ask in a frightened tone, "Is the HUC gone for the night?"

Thank you, HUCs, for all that you do.

To all the emergency department technicians, aka "techs": Whereas the HUCs are the do-it-all folks for non-clinical functions, techs are the Swiss Army knives in the clinical realm. Need an ECG done, a splint put on, blood drawn, POCT (point-of-care testing) run, assistance "road-testing" a patient (making sure they can safely walk on their own to ensure they can go home), some crackers and juice or some chest compressions? Where's the tech?

That's a partial list, by the way. Hospital administrators don't want to hear this, but HUCs and techs are vastly underpaid.

Thank you, techs, for all that you do.

To the APCs, Advanced Practice Clinicians—the Nurse Practitioners and Physician Assistants: I have had the pleasure of working with some outstanding APCs, medical professionals with advanced degrees and training that are employed in most ERs across the country. Your skill set and expertise are appreciated by emergency physicians everywhere.

Thank you, APCs, for all that you do.

Now, to some of my favorite people in the entire world. To emergency nurses... what can I say? I tried to convey my appreciation in letters to the editor of the Journal of Emergency Nursing in 2004 and again in 2014, but several years into the third decade of my career now, I must say that I have never appreciated you or relied on you more. Your job is one of the toughest in the country.

Thank you for saving my butt countless times by double-checking my orders, or by ordering something I didn't think of that led us down the correct path. Thank you for your gentle (and sometimes more direct) suggestions, and for your leading questions because you knew exactly what needed to happen. Thank you for your patience, endurance and tolerance. Thank you for your dark sense of humor, for lightening the mood when the whole team needed it, and for being brave enough to shed a tear when no other response seemed appropriate. For everything you do, and for being the best teammates imaginable, you have my eternal gratitude. If there is a Heaven, I know that ER nurses have a special place in it. For now, you'll have to settle for a very special place in my heart.

Thank you, ER nurses, for all that you do.

To my fellow emergency physicians, my brothers and sisters in arms, I wish I had the words to express the breadth and depth of my admiration.

If you tell me you're an ER doc, I can make several assumptions about you. You work and play well with others, maybe better than any other doctors on the planet. You're the best problem solvers. You're adaptable and flexible. Your bullshit meter is a finely tuned instrument that allows you to get to the crux of a problem and fix it quickly.

You're tough: physically, mentally and emotionally. You ignore unfavorable conditions as if they didn't exist. I recall trying to suture an occipital scalp laceration, a cut on the back of the head, on an elderly female during residency when a surgeon asked me why I didn't just turn her over on her stomach to make my work easier. The thought hadn't occurred to me. It seemed to me that such a position would make the patient uncomfortable. If one of us was going to be uncomfortable, it should be me.

I've intubated patients on the side of a road in the dark, beside a lake, in a helicopter, and unexpectedly in some of the smallest rooms in the ER. You've all done similar things. Your comfort doesn't even factor into the equation. What does the patient need? That's all that matters to you.

You have the patience of Job and the bladder capacity of an elephant (I chose elephant because my Google search said that an elephant's bladder can hold nearly 5 gallons of fluid, yet it can pee as quickly as a cat—sounds about right). You have extremely selective hearing, able to filter out screaming babies, agitated psych patients and a plethora of alarms and ringing phones.

You sacrifice a lot to serve your fellow human beings. You give up nights, weekends and holidays with your families, as all health care workers do. When someone asks, "How was your day?" at the dinner table, your answer often makes one or more listeners at the table lose their appetites, which makes no sense to you.

Chances are high that you've puked in the bathroom at work, probably more than once. I remember telling my wife that I had thrown up at work. By that time, she was conditioned enough to my career that what surprised and grossed her out most wasn't the fact I was vomiting at work, rather that I was on my hands and knees on the floor in the ER bathroom. Disgusting! On the level of "it's kind of insane and probably a bad idea to work that way," ER doctors should call in sick a lot more often than you do, but I still admire your fortitude.

Odds are even better that you've cried somewhere at work, maybe off in a dark corner, or in the ambulance bay, likely by yourself without anyone knowing. You've witnessed things that would provide fodder for months of therapy for mere mortals, yet you cope as best you can in the moment and keep pushing to care for the next patient.

You put up with a tremendous amount of BS from more people and systems than you can count, yet you embody the principle of FIDO (Fuck It Drive On).

You work in the most difficult environment in civilized medicine, bar none. You don't just turn lemons into lemonade—you make lemon chiffon pie, lemon tarts, lemon bars, and when you need to, you make lemon drops.

Are you perfect? Nope—that's why you're my favorite people. I'm not either. I don't even know what perfect would look like, but I know how hard it is to do what you do, especially to do it as well as you do. I understand how things sometimes get missed, or why you were pushed past your breaking point, if only momentarily. I see how hard you try. I feel how much it means to you.

I am privileged to share your profession. I am humbled to be counted among you. I love you for what you do and who you are.

There may be some jobs that are cooler. Fighter pilot comes to mind. Astronaut. Consigliere. ER doc is a pretty good one, though.

Thank you, my fellow ER docs, for all that you do.

Lastly, to our patients, without whom we'd all have made a lot of effort for nothing, be confident in knowing that should you or someone you love ever need to go to the emergency room, you will find a group of people who are highly trained, incredibly skilled, and deeply dedicated to helping and serving others. The interaction we offer you will be nothing if not a human one. If you try to BS us, we might sound annoyed. If we're in the middle of a case like one of the encounters I've described herein, I hope you'll understand if you have to wait a little longer. I can promise you this, though: if you come to the ER with a life-threatening condition, we'll leave it all on the field. For better or worse, your story may stick with us for the rest of our lives. Humanity is also a team sport.

Should you ever find yourself in a moment of medical crisis, fearing you or someone you love is seriously injured or ill, don't hesitate to come to us. As they say every time you call anyone who works in health care for any reason whatsoever, "If you are suffering from a life-threatening emergency, please hang up and call 911." They'll bring you to the ER.

Otherwise, just look for the red and white sign that says, "Emergency". We'll be ready for you.

About the Author

Reggie Duling was born and raised in Toledo, Ohio, the blue-collar home of Jeep, Libbey, Owens Corning and other icons of manufacturing that represent the best of the American work ethic. Reggie's parents always told him that he might not be smarter than the next person, but he could always outwork them, a lesson he employed to win multiple Soldier of the Year competitions while serving in the Army.

He obtained a BA in Philosophy at the University of Toledo, his medical degree at The Ohio State University, and completed emergency medicine residency at St. Vincent Mercy Medical Center and The Toledo Hospital, where he was chosen by his peers to serve as Chief Resident.

He is most proud of three professional achievements: the fact that he's always been a pit doc first and foremost, and that he has had the privilege of serving as President/CEO of MREP and EEP, two incredible groups of outstanding ER docs. His pride is rooted not in the titles, but rather in the fact that he was chosen and trusted by his peers to serve them.

Reggie lives in Washington with his soulmate and wife, Janina, and his three amazing children, Logan, Carson, and Jessica, as well as two of man's best friends, Cody and Ollie.

In his free time, Reggie enjoys jamming with his garage band and co-hosts *The Game, a Michigan and Ohio State Podcast*. He's tried his hand at woodworking, is a lifelong learner and holds tight to a few core beliefs.

His dad taught him the first, that "can't" shouldn't be in a man's vocabulary. The second is the wisdom of

Teddy Roosevelt: that the credit belongs to the man who is actually in the arena. The third is his belief that a person should not be measured by successes and failures, rather by the constant pursuit of improvement. If you never fail, you're not pushing yourself hard enough.

Made in the USA
Middletown, DE
05 November 2022

14175102R00129